MEDICAL
INTELLIGENCE
UNIT

THE IMMUNE FUNCTIONS OF EPIDERMAL LANGERHANS CELLS

MEDICAL
INTELLIGENCE
UNIT

THE IMMUNE FUNCTIONS OF EPIDERMAL LANGERHANS CELLS

Heidrun Moll, Ph.D.

University of Würzburg
Würzburg, Germany

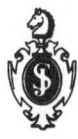

Springer-Verlag Berlin Heidelberg GmbH

MEDICAL INTELLIGENCE UNIT
THE IMMUNE FUNCTIONS OF EPIDERMAL LANGERHANS CELLS

International Copyright © 1995 Springer-Verlag Berlin Heidelberg
Originally published by Springer-Verlag Berlin Heidelberg New York in 1995
Softcover reprint of the hardcover 1st edition 1995

International ISBN 978-3-662-22499-1

Library of Congress Cataloging-in-Publication Data

The immune function of epidermal Langerhans cells / [edited by]
    Heidrun Moll
        p. cm. — (Medical intelligence unit)
    Includes bibliographical references and index.
    ISBN 978-3-662-22499-1   ISBN 978-3-662-22497-7 (eBook)
    DOI 10.1007/978-3-662-22497-7
    1. Langerhans cells 2. Skin—Immunology. I. Moll, Heidrun, 1957-   . II. Series.
        [DNLM: 1. Langerhans cell immunology. QW 568 I3143 1995]
QR185.8.L35146 1995
612.7'9—dc20
DNLM/DLC   95-14342
for Library of Congress   CIP

PUBLISHER'S NOTE

R.G. Landes Company publishes five book series: *Medical Intelligence Unit, Molecular Biology Intelligence Unit, Neuroscience Intelligence Unit, Tissue Engineering Intelligence Unit* and *Biotechnology Intelligence Unit.* The authors of our books are acknowledged leaders in their fields and the topics are unique. Almost without exception, no other similar books exist on these topics.

Our goal is to publish books in important and rapidly changing areas of medicine for sophisticated researchers and clinicians. To achieve this goal, we have accelerated our publishing program to conform to the fast pace in which information grows in biomedical science. Most of our books are published within 90 to 120 days of receipt of the manuscript. We would like to thank our readers for their continuing interest and welcome any comments or suggestions they may have for future books.

Deborah Muir Molsberry
Publications Director
R.G. Landes Company

CONTENTS

EDITOR

Heidrun Moll, Ph.D.
Research Center for Infectious Diseases
University of Würzburg
Würzburg, Germany
Chapter 10

CONTRIBUTORS

Paul R. Bergstresser, M.D.
Department of Dermatology
University of Texas Southwestern
  Medical Center
Dallas, Texas, U.S.A.
Chapter 8

Christine Blank, M.Sc.
Research Center for Infectious
  Diseases
University of Würzburg
Würzburg, Germany
Chapter 10

Anne-Sophie Charbonnier, M.A.
Peau Humaine et Immunité
Hôpital Edouard Herriot
Lyon, France
Chapter 11

Marie Cumberbatch, B.Sc., M.Sc.
Zeneca Central Toxicology
  Laboratory
Macclesfield
Cheshire, United Kingdom
Chapter 7

Pascale Delorme, Ph.D.
Peau Humaine et Immunité
Hôpital Edouard Herriot
Lyon, France
Chapter 11

Karin Demleitner, M.Sc.
Institute of Immunology
Johannes Gutenberg-University
Mainz, Germany
Chapter 6

Claude Desgranges, Ph.D.
Hépatite, SIDA et Rétrovirus Humains
Lyon, France
Chapter 11

Colette Dezutter-Dambuyant, Ph.D.
Peau Humaine et Immunité
Hôpital Edouard Herriot
Lyon, France
Chapter 11

Nathalie Dusserre, Ph.D.
Peau Humaine et Immunité
Hôpital Edouard Herriot
Lyon, France
Chapter 11

Andreas Eggert
Department of Dermatology
University of Würzburg
Würzburg, Germany
Chapter 3

CONTRIBUTORS

Alexander H. Enk, M.D.
Clinical Research Unit
Dermatology Department
Johannes Gutenberg-University
Mainz, Germany
Chapter 4

Marie-Madeleine Fiers
Peau Humaine et Immunité
Hôpital Edouard Herriot
Lyon, France
Chapter 11

Stefanie Flohé, M.Sc.
Research Center for Infectious
 Diseases
University of Würzburg
Würzburg, Germany
Chapter 10

Stephan Grabbe, M.D.
Department of Dermatology
University of Münster
Münster, Germany
Chapter 9

Richard D. Granstein, M.D.
Cutaneous Biology Research Center
Department of Dermatology
Massachusetts General Hospital
Harvard Medical School
Charlestown, Massachusetts, U.S.A.
Chapter 9

Kayo Inaba, Ph.D.
Department of Zoology
Faculty of Science
Kyoto University
Kyoto, Japan
Chapter 1

Eckhart Kämpgen, M.D.
Department of Dermatology
University of Würzburg
Würzburg, Germany
Chapter 3

Stephen I. Katz, M.D., Ph.D.
Dermatology Branch
National Cancer Institute
National Institute of Health
Bethesda, Maryland, U.S.A.
Chapter 4

Ian Kimber, B.Sc., M.Sc., Ph.D.
Zeneca Central Toxicology
 Laboratory
Macclesfield
Cheshire, United Kingdom
Chapter 7

Franz Koch, Ph.D.
Department of Dermatology
University of Innsbruck
Innsbruck, Austria
Chapter 3

Frits Koning, Ph.D.
Immunohematology and Bloodbank
University Hospital
Leiden, The Netherlands
Chapter 5

François Mallet, Ph.D.
Laboratoires Bio/Mérieux
Ecole Nationale Supérieure de Lyon
Lyon, France
Chapter 11

Alexandra Marx
Institute of Immunology
Johannes Gutenberg-University
Mainz, Germany
Chapter 6

CONTRIBUTORS

Maria Mehlig, M.Sc.
Institute of Immunology
Johannes Gutenberg-University
Mainz, Germany
Chapter 6

A. Mieke Mommaas, Ph.D.
Laboratory for Electron Microscopy
University Hospital Leiden
Leiden, The Netherlands
Chapter 5

Ursula Neiß, M.Sc.
Institute of Immunology
Johannes Gutenberg-University
Mainz, Germany
Chapter 6

Konrad Reske, Ph.D.
Institute of Immunology
Johannes Gutenberg-University
Mainz, Germany
Chapter 6

Nikolaus Romani, Ph.D.
Department of Dermatology
University of Innsbruck
Innsbruck, Austria
Chapter 3

Christoph Scheicher, Ph.D.
Institute of Immunology
Johannes Gutenberg-University
Mainz, Germany
Chapter 6

Daniel Schmitt, Ph.D.
Peau Humaine et Immunité
Hôpital Edouard Herriot
Lyon, France
Chapter 11

Gerold Schuler, M.D.
Department of Dermatology
University of Innsbruck
Innsbruck, Austria
Chapter 1, 3

Ralph M. Steinman, M.D.
Laboratory of Cellular Physiology
   and Immunology
The Rockefeller University
New York, New York, U.S.A.
Chapter 1

Georg Stingl, M.D.
Division of Immunology, Allergy
   and Infectious Diseases
Department of Dermatology
University of Vienna Medical School
Vienna, Austria
Chapter 2

Dirk Strunk, M.D.
Division of Immunology, Allergy
   and Infectious Diseases
Department of Dermatology
University of Vienna Medical School
Vienna, Austria
Chapter 2

Akira Takashima, M.D., Ph.D.
Department of Dermatology
University of Texas Southwestern
   Medical Center
Dallas, Texas, U.S.A.
Chapter 8

Catherine Tsagarakis, M.A.
Laboratoire d'Immunopathologie
Ecole Nationale Vétérinaire de Lyon
Marcy l'Etoile, France
Chapter 11

PREFACE

Epidermal Langerhans cells, a constituent of the skin immune system, have a spectrum of different functions with implications that extend far beyond the skin. They have the potential to capture allergens and infectious agents, they stimulate vigorous immune responses and they display migratory properties that equip them with the unique possibility to communicate between skin and lymph nodes. Langerhans cells are considered to play a pivotal role in infectious diseases such as AIDS, in allergy, autoimmunity, chronic inflammatory reactions, tumor rejection, transplantation and in effects caused by ultraviolet radiation.

The contributions to this book reflect this diversity, embracing various aspects of the current research on the immune functions of Langerhans cells and other dendritic cells. The topics range from the molecular characterization of Langerhans-cell function to the development of strategies that may allow the use of these cells in clinical medicine. In particular, the elucidation of mechanisms of antigen processing and presentation, the knowledge of which has developed explosively, and the tremendous advances in the generation of Langerhans cells in vitro for potential application in immunotherapy are described. It is hoped that this collection of articles stimulates continued research on the immunological functions of cutaneous dendritic cells.

CHAPTER 1

INTRODUCTION:
CUTANEOUS DENDRITIC CELLS:
DISTINCTIVE ANTIGEN-PRESENTING
CELLS FOR EXPERIMENTAL MODELS
AND DISEASE STATES

Ralph M. Steinman, Kayo Inaba, Gerold Schuler

Cutaneous dendritic cells, which include the Langerhans cells (LC) of the epidermis as well as their counterparts in the dermis and cutaneous lymph, have provided a rich area for investigative dermatology and immunology. The important starting points were the findings that LC are bone marrow-derived and have many properties of white blood cells such as binding of immune complexes, expression of major histocompatibility complex (MHC) class II products, and presentation of antigens to T cells. Much of this work is discussed in a compendium, Epidermal Langerhans Cells, edited by Dr. G. Schuler and published by CRC Press, Boca Raton, FL in 1991. Here, Dr. Heidrun Moll assembles an important series of articles that cover the latest, most timely developments.

Two themes are interwoven in this volume. One theme relates to LC as antigen-presenting cells (APC) for experimental models. This is emphasized by articles on the localization of MHC class II in LC (chapter 5 by Mommaas and Koning), the presentation of proteins (chapter 6 by Neiß et al), the alterations mediated by

The Immune Functions of Epidermal Langerhans Cells, edited by Heidrun Moll.
© 1995 R.G. Landes Company.

ultraviolet light (chapter 8 by Bergstresser and Takashima), and the critical regulation of LC at the level of cytokines (chapter 3 by Kämpgen et al, and chapter 7 by Kimber and Cumberbatch). The second theme is the importance of LC in clinical medicine. This is developed in chapters on contact allergy and tolerance (chapter 4 by Enk and Katz), tumor immunology (chapter 9 by Grabbe and Granstein), immune therapy (chapter 2 by Strunk and Stingl), cutaneous leishmaniasis (chapter 10 by Moll et al) and infection with human immunodeficiency virus (HIV) (chapter 11 by Dezutter-Dambuyant et al).

These two themes—cutaneous dendritic cells as APC for model antigens and disease states—in turn raise two questions that may already have occurred to the reader. First, why bother to study cutaneous dendritic cells as APC in experimental models? After all, these cells are neither abundant nor easy to isolate. Why not study more abundant and accessible APC like human blood monocytes, mouse peritoneal macrophages, or B cells from human blood and mouse spleen? Second, why are cutaneous dendritic cells central to such broad topics as infectious disease and tumor immunity? We will pursue answers to these questions in this introduction.

CUTANEOUS DENDRITIC CELLS
AS MEMBERS OF THE DENDRITIC CELL SYSTEM

The answer to the first question, "why bother to study cutaneous dendritic cells as APC in experimental models," is that these cells are not simply antigen-presenting cells. Instead, dendritic cells are highly specialized relative to other APC, with literally dozens of accessory functions to stimulate T cells. Cutaneous dendritic cells are the best-studied, peripheral outpost of the dendritic cell system and have been used to unravel several of its features. What are the differences in general terms between an APC and an accessory dendritic cell (Fig. 1.1)?

"Antigen presentation" refers to the many steps whereby a cell generates complexes between an antigen-presenting MHC molecule and a portion of the native antigen, either a peptide fragment of the antigen or a larger polypeptide superantigen (Fig. 1.1). Antigen presentation generates the ligand that is recognized by the clonotypic T cell receptor. As a result, antigen presentation underlies immunologic specificity, be it for immunity or tolerance. However, all cells that express class I and II MHC products seem ca-

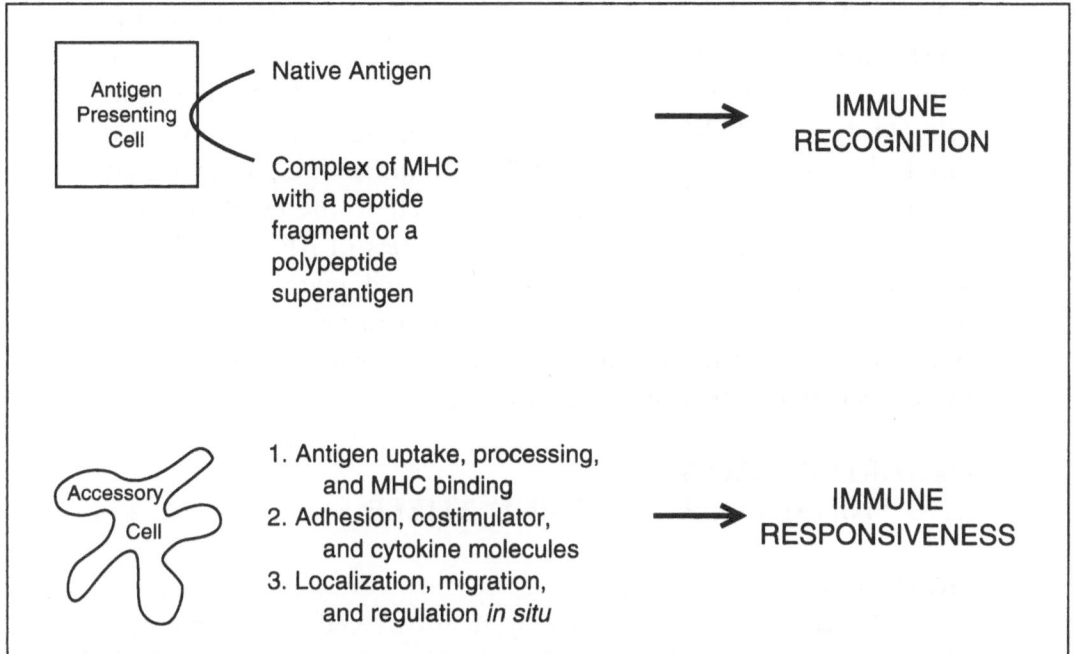

Fig. 1.1. Two distinct aspects of T cell mediated function.

pable of presenting antigens, since presentation is the only clear function of the polymorphic products of the MHC (in man, class I HLA-A, B, C and class II HLA-DR, DQ, DR; in mouse, H-2K, D, L and I-A, E, respectively).

Antigen presentation has been studied most extensively using clonal populations, either immortalized T–T hybridomas or chronically stimulated T cell lines and clones. Antigen presentation, while essential, is far from the only element of T-dependent responsiveness, be it immunity or tolerance. Instead, there are many accessory functions that play a role, particularly when one considers responses by infrequent clones of quiescent T cells in situ. These accessory functions help explain the potency of dendritic cells as APC as well as their capacity to stimulate naive T cells, including T cells in situ.

The functions of dendritic cells, in skin and in other tissues, fall into three broad categories of events or signals (Fig. 1.1): (1) "signal one," i.e., factors that influence the efficacy of antigen capture, processing and association with MHC products; (2) "signal two," i.e., factors that work together with antigen presentation and include (i) adhesion molecules that mediate the binding of

APC to T cells, (ii) costimulator molecules that help signal the T cells to make lymphokines or cytolytic molecules and (iii) soluble products or cytokines that instruct the T cell to form T helper cells of type 1 (Th1) vs. Th2 lymphokines (interferon-γ vs. interleukin (IL) 4 and IL-5); (3) "signal three," i.e., factors that allow immunity to develop in situ and include the cytokines and migration pathways that enable specific subsets of APC and T cells to be mobilized and to interact within defined anatomic compartments. We will review these three broad areas of accessory function, which according to current information can be expressed by LC as well as dendritic cells from other tissues.

DENDRITIC CELLS AND SIGNALS ONE, TWO AND THREE

SIGNAL ONE

The specializations exhibited by dendritic cells are numerous. Many were first identified in skin.

1. Dendritic cells express high levels of antigen-presenting molecules, especially MHC class II. On average, mouse epidermal LC have more than 10^6 binding sites for antibodies to MHC class II (I-A),[1] while human blood dendritic cells have a comparable number of binding sites for the superantigen, staphylococcal enterotoxin A.[2]

2. Paradoxically, dendritic cells do not appear to need large amounts of presented antigen to stimulate quiescent T cells. The amount of bound superantigen that is required for dendritic cells to stimulate naive T cells from human blood is estimated to be as low as a few hundred MHC-superantigen complexes per cell.[2] In the case of MHC class I, there are recent findings that dendritic cells can present nonreplicating forms of influenza virus as efficiently as live replicating virus (Bender et al, submitted).

3. Dendritic cells appear capable of retaining antigen in a form that is immunogenic for T cells for prolonged periods, for at least days in vitro[2,3] and in situ.[4,5] This retention likely results from the two features that were just mentioned, i.e., dendritic cells may be able to generate high levels of signal one (MHC-peptide complexes)

that turn over very slowly, yet only very small amounts of signal one are needed for the dendritic cell to be effective. An example of antigen retention is reviewed here by Moll et al, who observe the persistence of *Leishmania* in dendritic cells for weeks. However, it must be remembered that immunogenic peptides also could persist for long periods without being able to detect the original native antigen.

4. Dendritic cells can synthesize MHC class II and the associated invariant chain at high rates. When LC are isolated from mouse epidermis, the cells express within 14 hours close to 10^6 newly synthesized (i.e., cyclohex-imide-sensitive) I-A molecules,[6,7] and when LC are labeled with ^{35}S-methionine, the incorporation into MHC class II and invariant chain polypeptides is intense.[3,8,9] Biosynthesis is important, because according to current evidence, peptides most readily access MHC molecules when (1) newly synthesized MHC class II enters the endocytic system, (2) the associated invariant chain is proteolyzed and (3) the peptides have access to "empty" MHC class II, peptide-binding grooves.

5. Dendritic cells seem to have a distinct endocytic vacu-olar system that is relatively rich in multivesicular and multilamellar bodies.[10-12] Recent electron microscopic studies from Kleijmeer et al,[13] and from Mommaas and Koning in this volume, indicate that these vacuoles are rich in MHC class II and may function similarly to "CIIV's" (Class II MHC Vesicles) that have been isolated from antigen-presenting cell lines.[14,15] CIIVs represent a meeting place for endocytosed antigens, certain lysosomal proteases and newly synthesized MHC class II molecules from which invariant chains have been proteolyzed. In these vacuoles, peptide loading of MHC class II is thought to occur, followed by recycling to the cell surface.

6. The regulation of MHC class II biosynthesis and the vacuolar system is different for dendritic cells relative to other leukocytes. The simple isolation of LC from skin is associated with a marked, T cell independent upregulation of MHC class II.[3,6,8] Within 14 hours,

biosynthesis stops and acidic endocytic vacuoles diminish. Regulatory mechanisms remain undetermined. Nevertheless, dendritic cells seem poised to rapidly upregulate MHC class II upon minimal provocation, e.g., release from the epidermis into tissue culture,[6] transplantation,[16] application of contact allergens.[17]

7. Dendritic cells may have specialized mechanisms for antigen capture. For soluble molecules, Fc receptor-mediated endocytosis of immunoglobulins (Ig)[18] and macropinocytosis of tetanus toxin[19] already have been described. For particulates, dendritic cells can take up small numbers of certain particulates (mycobacteria, zymosan, *Leishmania*),[20,21] although only at certain periods in their life history (see below).

All of these features in "signal one" biology may contribute to the fact that dendritic cells are so potent, i.e., relatively low doses of cells and of antigen[4,22] are needed to stimulate T-cell responses.

Signal Two

There are several membrane "molecular couples" that influence the APC T cell interaction. Most are expressed by dendritic cells, i.e., CD11/CD18 integrins, intercellular adhesion molecules (ICAMs), lymphocyte function-associated antigen 3 (LFA-3), heat-stable antigen, CD40 and both CD80/B7-1 and CD86/B7-2 (Table 1.1). These couples may serve adhesive and/or costimulatory roles, mediating the binding of dendritic cells to T cells and/or the stimulation of specific intercellular pathways. Dendritic cells can express several of these accessory molecules simultaneously and at relatively high levels.[23-26] These molecules also can be upregulated very rapidly in a T cell independent manner.[26]

The observations of Bhardwaj et al[2] illustrate the potency of "signal two" in dendritic cells relative to other APC. They pulsed B cells with high concentrations of superantigen to achieve levels of bound "signal one" that were comparable to dendritic cells that had been exposed to low doses of superantigen. They found that one still requires a 30-fold lower dose of dendritic cells than B cells to stimulate equivalent levels of DNA synthesis (^{3}H-thymidine uptake).

With respect to cytokines that could underlie the ability of dendritic cells to stimulate T cells, the two main candidates are

Table 1.1. Accessory molecules that are prominently expressed on cutaneous dendritic cells

Dendritic cell	T-cell counter receptor
ICAM-1 (CD54)	LFA-1 (CD11a)
ICAM-3 (CD50)	LFA-1 (CD11a)
LFA-3 (CD58)	CD2
B7-1 (CD80)	CD28 and CTLA-4
B7-2 (CD86)	CD28 and CTLA-4
Heat-stable antigen	not known
MHC class I	CD8
MHC class II	CD4
CD40	CD40 ligand

IL-1β[17, 27] and IL-12,[28] which have been found to be abundant at the mRNA level.

The "signal two" area needs a good deal more work in the context of LC and other dendritic cells. Do dendritic cells express "signal-two" molecules that are distinct from other APC, or does the potent accessory function simply relate to the amount and regulation of "signal two"? Nonetheless, what is known at this time helps explain the physiologic fact that dendritic cells efficiently form multicellular clusters with T cells that are specific for the antigens and superantigens being presented; within these aggregates, extensive T cell activation (lymphokine production, cytolytic T cell development, T cell growth) takes place.

SIGNAL THREE

The in situ properties of dendritic cells represent the major qualitative differences between these cells and other APC. The location of dendritic cells in external epithelia like skin, mucous membranes and airway epithelium seems specific for this cell type in the steady state. For LC, the expression of epithelial, or E-, cadherin has been implicated in epithelial localization.[29] The capacity of cutaneous dendritic cells to move into afferent lymph, and thereby to the draining lymph node, is also distinctive both in the steady state (reviewed in ref. 30) and following such stimuli as transplantation and contact allergy (see below). Finally, dendritic cells can home via the lymph or the blood stream to the T cell areas of lymph node and spleen,[31,32] thereby gaining access to quiescent T cells that recirculate through the T dependent regions. These properties of dendritic cells likely explain another facet of their physiology, their capacity to prime or sensitize T dependent immune responses in situ.[4,5,33-35]

COORDINATING SIGNALS ONE, TWO AND THREE: MATURATION AND MIGRATION

LC have been analyzed in many of the above studies of signals one, two and three on dendritic cells. Yet there are two areas where the skin (epidermis, dermis and cutaneous lymphatics) stands out relative to other tissues. The first is the phenomenon of *"maturation."* This refers to the fact that cutaneous dendritic cells in situ need not be immunostimulatory accessory cells. Instead, freshly isolated LC need to differentiate in many ways (morphology, surface phenotype, function) before they resemble the stimulatory dendritic cells from lymphoid tissues and lymph.[1] At the level of "signal one," freshly isolated LC contain many acidic endosomes,[10] actively synthesize MHC class I and II (and invariant chain) molecules,[3,6,8] express moderate levels of Fc receptors[36] and functional receptors for other particulates,[20] and efficiently capture protein antigens.[37,38] Each of these features is then downregulated over a one to three-day period in culture. Acidic endosomes decrease in number, biosynthesis of MHC products is virtually extinguished, Fc and other phagocytic receptors diminish and presentation of protein antigens is reduced by one to two logarithms. At the level of "signal two," LC in situ express ICAM-3, but only in culture are many of the other accessory molecules and cytokines upregulated, including IL-1β, ICAM-1, LFA-3, CD40, CD80/B7-1, and especially CD86/B7-2.[23,24,26,39] In other words, freshly isolated LC are specialized for generating "signal one" while cultured LC are specialized for delivering "signal two" (Table 1.2).

The control of these maturation events is not worked out. IL-1β has been implicated in vivo.[17] This result is perplexing given the fact that IL-1α is inactive in vivo but shares a similar cell receptor with IL-1β. As reviewed in the article by Kämpgen et al, mouse LC have relatively abundant IL-1 type I receptors and receptors for granulocyte/macrophage colony-stimulating factor (GM-CSF),[40] raising the possibility that IL-1α (a major keratinocyte product) induces receptors for GM-CSF (another keratinocyte product), and the latter improves LC viability and function.[41,42] Comparable maturation events now are

Table 1.2. Maturation of Langerhans cells in culture

Property	0 - 12 hours	12 - 72 hours
Biosynthesis of MHC products, invariant chain	+++	–
Acidic endocytic vacuoles	+++	+
Fc receptors (CD32)	++	+
Protein presentation to primed T cells	+++	–
Adhesion and costimulator molecules	+ .	+++
IL-1 mRNA	+	++

evident in several tissues such as rat lung, mouse spleen, human blood and mouse heart and kidney. Of considerable interest are the recent studies of Sallusto and Lanzavecchia.[22] They appear to have "frozen" the antigen-capture mode of immature dendritic cells in long-term cultures of human blood cells that have been maintained in GM-CSF and IL-4. Tumor necrosis factor α (TNF-α), IL-1, CD40 ligand and lipopolysaccharide each can divert the cells from this actively endocytic mode and, at the same time, markedly downregulate the number of intracellular CIIVs.

The second area of dendritic cell biology in which the study of LC has been critical is that of *"migration,"* i.e., the specific routes that dendritic cells utilize to initiate T-dependent immunity. Silberberg-Sinakin et al noted typical LC in the afferent lymphatics of guinea pig skin to which a contact allergen had been applied.[43] Coupled with earlier ideas that epidermal LC acted as "reticuloepithelial traps" for contact allergens,[44] it seemed likely that contact allergens would move in association with LC via the lymphatics to the draining lymph node, thereby accounting for the need for intact lymphatics for sensitization to take place.[45] Several investigators have since isolated APC that bear contact allergens from draining lymph nodes and lymph.

In any case, Schuler's laboratory has considerable evidence, to date published only in an abstract form,[46] wherein contact allergens were compared to nonsensitizing chemicals. Only the allergens induced the migration of LC out of the epidermis and into the dermis. In the dermis, the LC aligned in "cords" and expressed abundant MHC class II molecules, as is typical of LC. By electron microscopy, these cords corresponded to afferent lymphatics and were full of LC.

Comparable migratory events occur in other contexts. Whenever cells in cutaneous afferent lymph have been studied, the frequency and flux of dendritic cells are high (reviewed in ref. 30). This steady-state migration of dendritic cells probably does *not* involve epidermal LC, since the turnover of the latter is slow; an origin from blood seems more likely. Nonetheless, during skin transplantation to either syngeneic or allogeneic recipients,[16] or following administration of endotoxin systemically,[47] at least two-thirds of the epidermal LC can migrate into the dermis to form "cords" of APC presumably in afferent lymphatics. The cells in these cords exhibit the upregulation of MHC class II and B7 costimulator molecules that is characteristic of mature LC.[16,39] The coupling of dendritic cell maturation and migration is unlikely to be limited to skin. In vascularized heart transplants, donor dendritic cells migrate via the blood to the spleen of the recipient.[48] If mature splenic dendritic cells or dendritic cells derived from proliferating progenitors are injected into an animal, APC are noted in the T cell areas of the draining lymphoid tissues.[31,49]

Cutaneous dendritic cells not only interact with naive T cells in the draining lymph node. LC also accumulate in the dermis in delayed-type hypersensitivity sites, which are a classical manifestation of prior T-cell priming or memory.

The molecular basis for dendritic cell migration in vivo is the subject of the articles by Enk and Katz, and Kimber and Cumberbatch. Cytokines like IL-1β[17] and TNF-α,[50,51] and adhesion molecules like ICAM-1 and LFA-1,[52] have been implicated. Perhaps these issues will be amenable to attack in organ culture. In explants of mouse and human skin (epidermis and dermis), dendritic cells literally emigrate from the skin into the culture medium over a one to three-day period. The emigrated cells have the morphology, phenotype and function of mature or highly stimulatory dendritic cells.[16,53]

It has been postulated that dendritic cell maturation and migration are pivotal to the onset of T cell mediated immunity.[1,16,37] Matzinger has written in some detail on this matter and refers to mature dendritic cells as "professional" APC because of the capacity to sensitize naive T cells.[54] She has proposed that the critical distinction between "self" and "nonself" does not necessarily relate to the origin of the antigen (self vs. foreign) but instead relates to the extent to which the antigen (self or foreign) is presented by dendritic cells that sense "danger." In effect, danger may operate by triggering the events of maturation and migration that have become evident from studies of cutaneous dendritic cells.

LANGERHANS CELLS IN MEDICINE

There are many areas of clinical medicine in which T lymphocytes play a critical role: allergy, transplantation, resistance to infection and tumors, autoimmunity and acquired immunodeficiency syndrome (AIDS). Much attention has been given to identifying disease-associated MHC polymorphisms and the corresponding presented antigens or superantigens. A variety of T cell suppressive therapies also have been tested. However, relatively little attention has been given to dendritic cells even though they express so many accessory properties that link the administration of antigen to T cell responsiveness. We will summarize some of the known relationships of dendritic cells to several clinical areas. In each case, cutaneous dendritic cells can provide the best access to a clinical problem that extends beyond the skin.

ALLERGY

This is being explored along two avenues. The first is delayed-type hypersensitivity such as contact allergy. Enk and Katz here summarize their innovative studies in which the cytokine IL-10 can modify LC so that tolerance rather than immunity ensues.[55] Perhaps IL-10 reduces expression of some costimulator(s) required for immunity. Kämpgen et al describe an additional route, i.e., LC that have been reared in the presence of TNF-α can induce anergy rather than immunity.[56] A second avenue entails IgE-mediated hypersensitivity. Two groups described the striking finding that IgE receptors are expressed by LC,[57,58] which likely accounts for the fact that IgE has been visualized in situ on epidermal LC in allergic individuals. Possibly IgE receptors allow trace levels of IgE to mediate the presentation of allergens to the Th2 type of helper cell. This in turn would produce the IL-4 that helps IgE antibody production and might induce inflammation.[59]

TRANSPLANTATION

An involvement of mature dendritic cells has been demonstrated during the induction of graft rejection[60] and probably in graft-versus-host disease as well.[61] Now attention is being given to another possibility, the use of donor-derived dendritic cells to induce tolerance.[62] These issues might be explored in skin much like the situation with contact allergens, i.e., it may be possible to alter dendritic cells so that tolerance rather than immunity is generated.

RESISTANCE TO INFECTION

Dendritic cells are implicated in the generation of resistance to cutaneous leishmaniasis.[21] As reviewed in the article by Moll et al, dendritic cells bearing these protozoa have been identified in the dermis and in the T cell areas of the draining lymph node. Other infectious agents have been offered to dendritic cells in culture, e.g., several viruses (particularly influenza)[63] and mycobacteria.[5] These are presented efficiently to antigen-specific CD4+ helper T cells and CD8+ killer T cells, but the induction of protective, anti-microbial immunity in situ remains to be shown.

RESISTANCE TO TUMORS

The skin and related mucous membranes figure prominently in several tumors for which immune therapies are envisaged. Melanoma and cervical cancer are the best examples, given the fact that several candidate antigens from melanomas and papilloma virus have been identified. To date, presentation of these antigens by dendritic cells has not been studied. However, the article by Grabbe and Granstein describes LC presentation of soluble antigens from a mouse sarcoma, primarily to CD4+ T cells. Recently, proliferating progenitors to dendritic cells have been identified in mouse and in man.[22,49,64-66] Therefore, more abundant populations of dendritic cells are available, and this should make it feasible to manipulate the immune system in situ, as discussed by Stingl and Strunk in this volume.

AUTOIMMUNITY

Examples in which autoimmunity has been studied from the perspective of dendritic cells include: rheumatoid arthritis, where the cells are abundant in synovial exudates; thyroiditis, where dendritic cells from affected mice can transfer autoimmunity; and psoriasis, where dendritic cells are abundant in both the epidermis (where there is an abnormal accumulation of CD8+ T cells) and dermis (where many CD4+ and CD8+ T cells are noted).

AIDS

Epidermal LC were one of the first sites in which CD4 expression by dendritic cells was noted.[67] Careful autopsy studies of epidermal LC from individuals afflicted with AIDS demonstrate a low frequency of LC that carry HIV-1 proviral DNA, typically around 1%.[68] Likewise, it has been difficult to demonstrate large-scale infection when HIV-1 is applied to purified LC in culture.[69] While some infection of LC with HIV-1 can take place, a special role of dendritic cells is more evident in the context of interacting T cells.

Pope et al, taking advantage of cells that emigrate from skin organ cultures,[53,70] recently identified a pathway whereby cutaneous dendritic cells can play a major role in HIV-1 infection.[69] They studied leukocytes that emigrate from skin explants. In addition to emigrating dendritic cells, many small αβ T cell receptor lymphocytes were noted. These T cells had the phenotype of memory cells (CD45RA[low], CD45RO[high], LFA-3[high]) and could form tight conjugates with the much larger dendritic cells. Comparable dendritic cell–T cell conjugates have been frequently described in analyses of afferent lymph from four different species including man. Because of the small size of these T cells (and lack of proliferation in culture),[53,69] the functional significance of the conjugates was unclear. When HIV-1 was added, however, an efficient productive and cytopathic infection ensued. This occurred with standard isolates like Ba-L and IIIB, and several recently-derived isolates of both syncytium-inducing and nonsyncytium-inducing phenotype. This permissive dendritic cell–T cell environment could have a physiological counterpart. Dendritic cell–T cell conjugates are normally found in lymph, and their numbers would increase whenever cutaneous dendritic cells are induced to mature and migrate. Given the presence of dendritic cells in the epithelia that cover all the organs involved in the sexual transmission of HIV-1 (vagina, anus, penis, pharynx), and given the predominance of T cells with the memory phenotype in the skin[71] and lymph,[72] it has been proposed that dendritic cell–T cell conjugates are a critical site for acute infection with HIV-1 and perhaps for the chronic production of virus and the loss of CD4[+] memory T cells.[69]

CONCLUSION

This book takes off from a rich literature on cutaneous dendritic cells. The development of this immunological perspective is summarized in many prior reviews, e.g., a recent compendium on Epidermal Langerhans Cells (ed. G. Schuler, CRC Press, Boca Raton, FL 1991). Now functional analyses at the cell and molecular levels are underway, as are studies in several clinical areas. These emerging topics, including the initial efforts to examine dendritic cells from the perspective of tolerance instead of immunity, are broadly sampled by the contributors to this volume.

To introduce this volume, we have chosen to emphasize two broad themes that permeate the contributions that follow. First, we outline reasons for studying LC as APC relative to other APC like macrophages and B lymphocytes. The specialized features of LC are summarized with respect to antigen presentation, to accessory molecules and to APC function in situ ("signals one, two and three," respectively). Second, we list areas in clinical immunology that might be impacted by further study of dendritic cells. Cutaneous dendritic cells, as represented by several articles within this volume, are an important part of the study of contact allergy, resistance to intracellular infections, tumor immunotherapy and HIV infection.

For both experimental and clinical studies, two important topics have been investigated in large part in the context of cutaneous dendritic cells. These are their maturation into typical immunostimulatory dendritic cells, primarily under the influence of cytokines like GM-CSF, and their migration along defined pathways in vivo so that contacts with T cells can develop. Further dissection of these maturation and migration events should bear fruit and will impinge upon clinical studies that analyze disease at the level of cutaneous dendritic cells.

ACKNOWLEDGMENTS

RS was supported by grants AI13013, AI07012 and AI24775 from the NIH. KI was supported by a grant from the Ministry of Education, Science and Culture of Japan (Grant-in-Aid for Science Research on Priority Areas and for Joint Research in International Scientific Research). GS was supported by the Austrian National Bank (Jubiläumsfonds project 4889) and the Austrian Science Foundation (SFB 207). The themes that are outlined in this article reflect the contributions of several longstanding colleagues: Jonathan Austyn, Nina Bhardwaj, Peter Fritsch, Christine Heufler, Lloyd Hoffman, Susumu Ikehara, Muneo Inaba, Franz Koch, Shigeru Muramatsu, Una O'Doherty, Melissa Pope, Nikolaus Romani, William Swiggard, Hella Stössel, James Young and the late Dr. Zanvil Cohn.

REFERENCES

1. Schuler G, Steinman RM. Murine epidermal Langerhans cells mature into potent immunostimulatory dendritic cells in vitro. J Exp Med 1985; 161:526-46.

2. Bhardwaj N, Young JW, Nisanian AJ et al. Small amounts of superantigen, when presented on dendritic cells, are sufficient to initiate T cell responses. J Exp Med 1993; 178:633-42.

3. Puré E, Inaba K, Crowley MT et al. Antigen processing by epidermal Langerhans cells correlates with the level of biosynthesis of major histocompatibility complex class II molecules and expression of invariant chain. J Exp Med 1990; 172:1459-69.

4. Inaba K, Metlay JP, Crowley MT et al. Dendritic cells pulsed with protein antigens in vitro can prime antigen-specific, MHC-restricted T cells in situ. J Exp Med 1990; 172:631-40.

5. Inaba K, Inaba M, Naito M et al. Dendritic cell progenitors phagocytose particulates, including Bacillus Calmette-Guerin organisms, and sensitize mice to mycobacterial antigens in vivo. J Exp Med 1993; 178:479-88.

6. Witmer-Pack MD, Valinsky J, Olivier W et al. Quantitation of surface antigens on cultured murine epidermal Langerhans cells: rapid and selective increase in the level of surface MHC products. J Invest Dermatol 1988; 90:387-94.

7. Shimada S, Caughman SW, Sharrow SO et al. Enhanced antigen-presenting capacity of cultured Langerhans cells is associated with markedly increased expression of Ia antigen. J Immunol 1987; 139:2551-5.

8. Kämpgen E, Koch N, Koch F et al. Class II major histocompatibility complex molecules of murine dendritic cells: synthesis, sialylation of invariant chain, and antigen processing capacity are down-regulated upon culture. Proc Natl Acad Sci USA 1991; 88:3014-8.

9. Scheicher C, Mehlig M, Zecher R et al. Dendritic cells from mouse bone marrow: in vitro differentiation using low doses of recombinant granulocyte-macrophage colony-stimulating factor. J Immunol Meth 1992; 154:253-64.

10. Stössel H, Koch F, Kämpgen E et al. Disappearance of certain acidic organelles (endosomes and Langerhans cell granules) accompanies loss of antigen processsing capacity upon culture of epidermal Langerhans cells. J Exp Med 1990; 172:1471-82.

11. Steinman RM, Kaplan G, Witmer MD et al. Identification of a novel cell type in peripheral lymphoid organs of mice. V. Purification of spleen dendritic cells, new surface markers, and maintenance in vitro. J Exp Med 1979; 149:1-16.

12. Girolomoni G, Cruz Jr PD, Bergstresser PR. Internalization and acidification of surface HLA-DR molecules by epidermal Langerhans cells: A paradigm for antigen processing. J Invest Dermatol 1990; 94:753.

13. Kleijmeer MJ, Oorschot VMJ, Geuze HJ. Human resident Langerhans cells display a lysosomal compartment enriched in MHC class II. J Invest Dermatol 1994; 103:516-23.

14. Tulp A, Verwoerd D, Dobberstein B et al. Isolation and characterization of the intracellular MHC class II compartment. Nature 1994; 369:120-6.

15. Amigorena S, Drake JR, Webster P et al. Transient accumulation of new class II MHC molecules in a novel endocytic compartment in B lymphocytes. Nature 1994; 369:113-20.

16. Larsen CP, Steinman RM, Witmer-Pack MD et al. Migration and maturation of Langerhans cells in skin transplants and explants. J Exp Med 1990; 172:1483-93.

17. Enk AH, Angeloni VL, Udey MC et al. An essential role for Langerhans cell-derived IL-1β in the induction of primary immune responses in skin. J Immunol 1993; 150:3698-704.

18. Zaghouani H, Steinman RM, Nonacs R et al. Efficient presentation of a viral T helper epitope expressed in the CDR3 region of a self immunoglobulin molecule. Science 1993; 259:224-7.

19. Sallusto F, Lanzavecchia A. Dendritic cells concentrate antigen in the class II compartment by macropinocytosis. Downregulation by cytokines and bacterial products. J Exp Med 1995; submitted.

20. Reis e Sousa C, Stahl PD, Austyn JM. Phagocytosis of antigens by Langerhans cells in vitro. J Exp Med 1993; 178:509-19.

21. Moll H, Fuchs H, Blank C, Röllinghoff M. Langerhans cells transport *Leishmania major* from the infected skin to the draining lymph node for presentation to antigen-specific T cells. Eur J Immunol 1993; 23:1595-1601.

22. Sallusto F, Lanzavecchia A. Efficient presentation of soluble antigen by cultured human dendritic cells is maintained by granulocyte/macrophage colony-stimulating factor plus interleukin 4 and downregulated by tumor necrosis factor α. J Exp Med 1994; 179:1109-18.

23. Romani N, Lenz A, Glassel H et al. Cultured human Langerhans cells resemble lymphoid dendritic cells in phenotype and function. J Invest Dermatol 1989; 93:600-9.

24. Teunissen MBM, Wormmeester J, Krieg SR et al. Human epidermal Langerhans cells undergo profound morphologic and phenotypical changes during in vitro culture. J Invest Dermatol 1990; 94:166-73.

25. Caux C, Vanbervlict B, Massacrier C et al. B70/B7-2 is identical to CD86 and is the major functional ligand for CD28 expressed on human dendritic cells. J Exp Med 1994; 180:1841-7.

26. Inaba K, Witmer-Pack M, Inaba M et al. The tissue distribution of the B7-2 costimulator in mice: abundant expression on dendritic cells in situ and during maturation. J Exp Med 1994; 180:1849-60.

27. Heufler C, Topar G, Koch F et al. Cytokine gene expression in murine epidermal cell suspensions: Interleukin 1 beta and macrophage inflammatory protein 1 alpha are selectively expressed in Langerhans cells but are differentially regulated in culture. J Exp Med 1992; 176:1221-6.

28. Heufler C, Topar G, Wysocka M et al. Dendritic cells are a source of interleukin-12. J Invest Dermatol 1994; 103:418(Abstract).

29. Tang A, Amagai M, Granger LG et al. Adhesion of epidermal

Langerhans cells to keratinocytes mediated by E-cadherin. Nature 1993; 361:82-5.

30. Steinman RM, Hoffman L, Pope M. Maturation and migration of cutaneous dendritic cells. J Invest Dermatol 1995; in press.

31. Austyn JM, Kupiec-Weglinski JW, Hankins DF et al. Migration patterns of dendritic cells in the mouse. Homing to T cell-dependent areas of spleen, and binding within marginal zone. J Exp Med 1988; 167:646-51.

32. Fossum S. Lymph-borne dendritic leukocytes do not recirculate, but enter the lymph node paracortex to become interdigitating cells. Scand J Immunol 1989; 27:97-105.

33. Havenith CEG, Breedijk AJ, Betjes MGH et al. T cell priming in situ by intratracheally instilled antigen-pulsed dendritic cells. Am J Resp Cell & Molec Biol 1993; 8:319-24.

34. Liu LM, MacPherson GG. Antigen acquisition by dendritic cells: Intestinal dendritic cells acquire antigen administered orally and can prime naive T cells "in vivo." J Exp Med 1993; 177:1299-1307.

35. Sornasse T, Flamand V, DeBecker G et al. Antigen-pulsed dendritic cells can efficiently induce an antibody response in vivo. J Exp Med 1992; 175:15-21.

36. Romani N, Inaba K, Puré E et al. A small number of anti-CD3 molecules on dendritic cells stimulate DNA synthesis in mouse T lymphocytes. J Exp Med 1989; 169:1153-68.

37. Romani N, Koide S, Crowley M et al. Presentation of exogenous protein antigens by dendritic cells to T cell clones: intact protein is presented best by immature, epidermal Langerhans cells. J Exp Med 1989; 169:1169-78.

38. Streilein JW, Grammer SF. In vitro evidence that Langerhans cells can adopt two functionally distinct forms capable of antigen presentation to T lymphocytes. J Immunol 1989; 143:3925-33.

39. Larsen CP, Ritchie SC, Hendrix R et al. Regulation of immunostimulatory function and costimulatory molecule (B7-1 and B7-2) expression on murine dendritic cells. J Immunol 1994; 152:5208-19.

40. Kämpgen E, Koch F, Heufler C et al. Understanding the dendritic cell lineage through a study of cytokine receptors. J Exp Med 1994; 179:1767-76.

41. Witmer-Pack MD, Olivier W, Valinsky J et al. Granulocyte/macrophage colony-stimulating factor is essential for the viability and function of cultured murine epidermal Langerhans cells. J Exp Med 1987; 166:1484-98.

42. Heufler C, Koch F, Schuler G. Granulocyte-macrophage colony-stimulating factor and interleukin-1 mediate the maturation of murine epidermal Langerhans cells into potent immunostimulatory dendritic cells. J Exp Med 1987; 167:700-5.

43. Silberberg-Sinakin I, Thorbecke GJ, Baer RL et al. Antigen-bearing Langerhans cells in skin, dermal lymphatics and in lymph nodes. Cell Immunol 1976; 25:137-51.

44. Shelley WB, Juhlin L. Langerhans cells form a reticuloepithelial trap for external contact allergens. Nature 1976; 261:46-7.
45. Frey JR, Wenk P. Experimental studies on the pathogenesis of contact eczema in the guinea pig. Intl Arch Allergy Appl Immunol 1957; 11:81-100.
46. Weinlich G, Sepp N, Koch F et al. Evidence that Langerhans cells rapidly disappear from the epidermis in response to contact sensitizers but not to tolerogens/ nonsensitizers. Arch Dermatol Res 1989; 281:556(Abstract).
47. Roake JA, Rao AS, Morris PJ et al. Dendritic cell loss from non-lymphoid tissues following systemic administration of lipopolysaccharide, tumour necrosis factor, and interleukin-1. Submitted.
48. Larsen CP, Morris PJ, Austyn JM. Migration of dendritic leukocytes from cardiac allografts into host spleens: a novel pathway for initiation of rejection. J Exp Med 1990; 171:307-14.
49. Inaba K, Steinman RM, Witmer-Pack M et al. Identification of proliferating dendritic cell precursors in mouse blood. J Exp Med 1992; 175:1157-67.
50. Cumberbatch M, Kimber I. Dermal tumour necrosis factor-alpha induces dendritic cell migration to draining lymph nodes, and possibly provides one stimulus for Langerhans' cell migration. Immunology 1992; 75:257-63.
51. MacPherson GG, Jenkins CD, Stein MJ et al. Endotoxin-mediated dendritic cell release from the intestine: Characterization of released dendritic cells and TNF dependence. J Immunol 1995; in press.
52. Ma J, Wang JH, Guo YJ et al. In vivo treatment with anti-ICAM and anti-LFA-1 antibodies inhibits contact sensitization-induced migration of epidermal Langerhans cells to regional lymph nodes. Cell Immunol 1994; 158:389-99.
53. Pope M, Betjes MGH, Hirmand H et al. Both dendritic cells and memory T lymphocytes emigrate from organ cultures of human skin and form distinctive dendritic-T cell conjugates. J Invest Dermatol 1995; in press.
54. Matzinger P. Tolerance, danger, and the extended family. Annu Rev Immunol 1994; 12:991-1045.
55. Enk AH, Saloga J, Becker D et al. Induction of hapten-specific tolerance by interleukin-10 in vivo. J Exp Med 1994; 179: 1397-1402.
56. Kämpgen E, Koch F, Enk AH et al. TNF alpha as well as IL-10 treated epidermal Langerhans cells induce antigen-specific tolerance yet by distinct mechanisms. Arch Dermatol Res 1995; in press.
57. Bieber T, de la Salle H, Wollenberg A et al. Human epidermal Langerhans cells express the high affinity receptor for immunoglobulin E (Fc epsilon). J Exp Med 1992; 175:1285-90.
58. Wang B, Rieger A, Kilgus O et al. Epidermal Langerhans cells from normal human skin bind monomeric IgE via Fc epsilon RI. J Exp Med 1992; 175:1353-65.

59. Muller KM, Jaunin F, Masouye I et al. Th2 cells mediate IL-4-dependent local tissue inflammation. J Immunol 1993; 150:5576-84.

60. Lechler RI, Batchelor JR. Restoration of immunogenicity to passenger cell-depleted kidney allografts by the addition of donor strain dendritic cells. J Exp Med 1982; 155:31-41.

61. Perreault C, Pelletier M, Belanger R et al. Persistence of host Langerhans cells following allogeneic bone marrow transplantation: possible relationship with acute graft-versus-host disease. Br J Haematol 1985; 60:253-60.

62. Starzl TE, Demetris AJ, Murase N et al. Cell migration, chimerism, and graft acceptance. Lancet 1992; 339:1579-82.

63. Bhardwaj N, Bender A, Gonzalez N et al. Influenza virus-infected dendritic cells stimulate strong proliferative and cytolytic responses from human CD8+ T cells. J Clin Invest 1994; 94:797-807.

64. Inaba K, Inaba M, Romani N et al. Generation of large numbers of dendritic cells from mouse bone marrow cultures supplemented with granulocyte-macrophage colony stimulating factor. J Exp Med 1992; 176:1693-1702.

65. Caux C, Dezutter-Dambuyant C, Schmitt D et al. GM-CSF and TNF-alpha cooperate in the generation of dendritic Langerhans cells. Nature 1992; 360:258-61.

66. Romani N, Gruner S, Brang D et al. Proliferating dendritic cell progenitors in human blood. J Exp Med 1994; 180:83-93.

67. Wood GS, Warner NL, Warnke RA. Anti-Leu-3/T4 antibodies react with cells of monocyte/macrophage and Langerhans lineage. J Immunol 1983; 131:212-6.

68. Cimarelli A, Zambruno G, Marconi A et al. Quantitation by competitive PCR of HIV-1 proviral DNA in epidermal Langerhans cells of HIV-infected patients. J Acquir Immune Defic Syndr 1994; 7:230-5.

69. Pope M, Betjes MGH, Romani N et al. Conjugates of dendritic cells and memory T lymphocytes from skin facilitate productive infection with HIV-1. Cell 1994; 78:389-98.

70. Richters CD, Hoekstra MJ, van Baare J et al. Isolation and chracterization of migratory human skin dendritic cells. Clin Exp Immunol 1994; 98:330-7.

71. Foster CA, Yokozeki H, Rappersberger K et al. Human epidermal T cells predominantly belong to the lineage expressing alpha/beta T cell receptor. J Exp Med 1990; 171:997-1013.

72. Mackay CR, Marston WL, Dudler L. Naive and memory T cells show distinct pathways of lymphocyte recirculation. J Exp Med 1990; 171:801-18.

CHAPTER 2

HUMAN LANGERHANS CELLS DERIVED FROM CD34+ BLOOD PRECURSORS: MODE OF GENERATION, PHENOTYPIC AND FUNCTIONAL ANALYSIS, AND EXPERIMENTAL AND CLINICAL APPLICABILITY

Dirk Strunk, Georg Stingl

INTRODUCTION

Epidermal Langerhans cells (LC) were originally described in 1868 as nerve cells within human skin.[1] After more than a century of speculations about their origin,[2,3] they were finally recognized to be hematopoietic cells as evidenced by their uniform expression of the panhematopoietic marker CD45 and by the presence of donor-derived phenotypic features on LC of H-2-disparate murine[4,5] and sex-mismatched human[6] bone marrow chimeras.

Within their epidermal residence, human LC can be identified as suprabasally located dendritic cells expressing CD1a, major histocompatibility complex (MHC) class II molecules, CD32, CD11b and Lag, and containing Birbeck granules (BG). Freshly isolated epidermal LC

---

effectively process exogenous soluble protein antigens but are only weak stimulators of naive T cells. During two to three days of in vitro culture with granulocyte/macrophage colony-stimulating factor (GM-CSF), LC downregulate the expression of several surface molecules, lose BG and reduce their antigen-processing capacity. In parallel, they upregulate MHC and costimulatory molecules to become potent immunostimulatory cells that resemble lymphoid dendritic cells in phenotype and function. Compelling evidence exists that LC function as sentinels of the immune system, capturing exogenous antigens in their local environment, carrying it via the afferent lymphatics to T cell dependent areas of the regional lymph nodes and, finally, presenting it at this site in an MHC-restricted fashion to naive T cells.[3,7,8]

The distinct accessory functions of LC and other dendritic cells in the generation of primary and secondary immune responses opened the attractive possibility to use these cells as "nature's adjuvant" in the therapy of cancer and infectious diseases.[9] Limitations in LC numbers, tedious isolation procedures, and a lack of culture conditions that maintain LC viability in vitro, have hampered progress in this field. A major step towards a resolution of these problems was the discovery that supernatants of mitogen-treated leukocytes contain factors that induce the outgrowth of dendritic cells in cultures of bone marrow cells in vitro.[10-12] Recently, GM-CSF alone or in combination with other cytokines has been shown to promote the generation of dendritic cells from precursors in bone marrow,[13-16] neonatal cord blood[17,18] and peripheral blood.[19-21] In our laboratory, we have developed a method for the generation of human LC from peripheral blood (Strunk et al, submitted for publication). This procedure involves the purification of hematopoietic progenitor cells (HPC), which, upon stimulation with the cytokines GM-CSF and tumor necrosis factor α (TNF-α) in the absence or presence of interleukin 4 (IL-4), give rise to BG-containing immunostimulatory LC.

GENERATION OF LANGERHANS CELLS FROM PERIPHERAL BLOOD

ISOLATION OF HEMATOPOIETIC PROGENITOR CELLS FROM PERIPHERAL BLOOD

Peripheral blood mononuclear cells (PBMC) from healthy adult individuals contain a minor population of CD34+ cells (approximately 0.1%), most of which are early committed HPC; in addition, there exists a minute fraction (<3% of the circulating CD34⁺ cells) of multipotent stem cells with self-renewal capacity.[22]

Flow cytometric analysis of circulating HPC by us (Strunk et al, submitted for publication) and others[22-24] has revealed that CD34⁺ HPC in peripheral blood of healthy adults express CD45 and MHC class I molecules and do not display the typical lineage markers of T lymphocytes (CD3, CD4, CD8), B lymphocytes (CD19, CD20), natural killer (NK) cells (CD56), monocytes (CD14, CD33), and erythrocytes (glycophorin A). They are also negative for several other leukocyte differentiation and activation antigens such as CD1a, CD1b, CD1c, CD11c, CD15, CD64, CD80, and HLA-DQ. Certain non-lineage-restricted molecules, including CD11b, Fc receptors (CD16, CD32), CD40, CD54, and CD58 can be detected on small sub-populations of CD34⁺ HPC. The majority of circulating HPC (>90%) express low levels of HLA-DR. We have also observed that approxi-mately 50% of circulating CD34⁺ cells react with the monoclonal antibody HECA-452 (Strunk et al, submitted for publication) which defines the cutaneous lymphocyte-associated antigen (CLA).[25,26] It will be interesting to see whether the expression of this antigen allows CD34⁺ HPC to home to the skin and, as a consequence, whether leukocyte differentiation can occur in this nonlymphoid organ.

There exist a number of methods for the isolation of CD34⁺ HPC. Most commonly used are cell separation techniques based on physical parameters, immunoadsorption, fluorescence-activated cell sorting, and combinations of these procedures. When applied to the isolation of CD34⁺ cells from normal peripheral blood, these meth-ods permit either high purity but low yield or vice versa.[22] We have developed a method which combines negative selection with HPC purification (Fig. 2.1). Depletion of T cells with sheep erythrocytes and monocytes by adhesion results in a tenfold enrichment of HPC without a loss in CD34⁺ cells. Positive selection with anti-CD34-coated paramagnetic beads and subsequent bead detachment allows for the efficient isolation of HPC from peripheral blood (yield: 40-95% of the CD34⁺ cells as compared to the starting population) with a purity of >95% (Strunk et al, submitted for publication).

DIFFERENTIATION OF CD34⁺ PROGENITORS INTO IMMUNOSTIMULATORY CD1A⁺ LANGERHANS CELLS

Survival and differentiation of isolated HPC in vitro are strictly dependent upon the presence of exogenous growth factors and/or

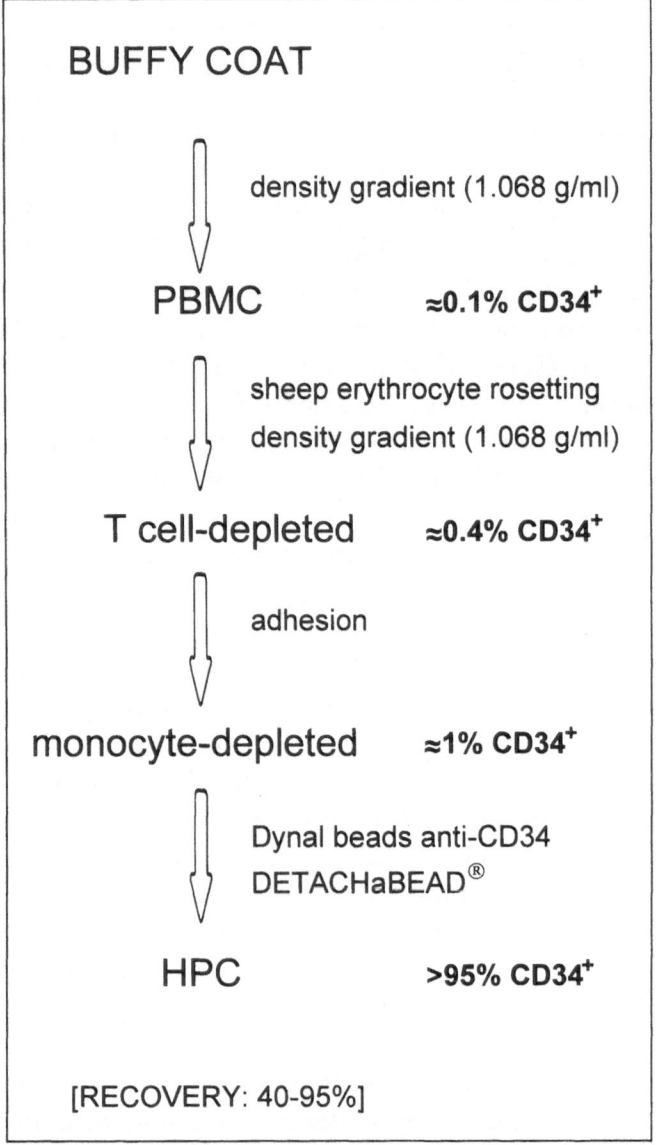

Fig. 2.1. Isolation of circulating CD34+ hematopoietic progenitor cells (HPC). Summarized in this scheme are the essential steps for the purification of CD34+ HPC from buffy coats prepared from peripheral blood of healthy adult volunteers. HPC, measured as % CD34-reactive cells, comprise approximately 0.1% of PBMC. After depletion of T cells and monocytes by rosetting with sheep red blood cells and adhesion, respectively, their concentration is increased to approximately 1% without a (non-) specific loss in CD34+ HPC. Cell sorting with anti-CD34-reactive magnetic beads (Dynal) allows for the effective and reproducible purification of circulating CD34+ HPC.

cytokines. Similar to what has been reported by Caux et al[18] for CD34⁺ cells from human cord blood, we found that CD34⁺ HPC from peripheral blood of healthy adults respond to stimulation with GM-CSF/TNF-α with a 15- to 42-fold (mean: 27-fold) multiplication of the starting cell number in the course of two weeks. During this period, clusters of dendritically shaped cells (DSC) can first be detected after four to five days of culture, and they increase in number and size during the following days. After two weeks of culture, three morphologically distinct populations of HPC-derived cells can be observed: (1) loosely adherent clusters of DSC (some of which are as large as 1 mm in diameter), (2) floating round or elongated nonadherent cells, and (3) adherent cells which morphologically resemble macrophages. Immuno-phenotyping of unfractionated GM-CSF/TNF-α-induced HPC-derived cells after two weeks of culture revealed that the majority (>95%) of the cells generated are CD68⁺ myeloid cells. Approximately one third of them are CD14⁺ cells and 10-15% of all viable cells express CD1a (Strunk et al, submitted for publication).

IL-4, known to inhibit the development of monocytes in bone marrow cultures,[27] acts in a comparable fashion in HPC cultures from peripheral blood. The addition of this cytokine to the combination of GM-CSF and TNF-α substantially reduces the cellular recovery compared to cultures with GM-CSF/TNF-α alone, abrogates the development of CD14⁺ cells almost completely but does not affect the generation of DSC clusters (Strunk et al, submitted for publication). Consequently, we found increased relative but not absolute numbers of CD1a⁺ cells in cultures stimulated with GM-CSF/TNF-α/IL-4 (Fig. 2.2).

Flow cytometric analysis revealed that all CD1a⁺ cells generated from circulating CD34⁺ HPC with GM-CSF and TNF-α are CD45⁺/MHC class I⁺ leukocytes that contain the CD68 antigen. In their majority they are CD4⁺, HLA-DR⁺, CD40⁺, CD80⁺, CD54⁺, and CLA⁺. Subpopulations of CD1a⁺ cells were found to express CD14 (50%), lymphocyte function-associated antigen 1 (LFA-1) and CD32 (35-40%), HLA-DQ and CD58 (approx. 20%), as well as CD1b, CD35, CD16 and CD64 (<10%). The in vitro generated CD1a⁺ cells did not stain with markers of mature T (CD3, CD8), B (CD19, CD20, CD21), or NK cells (CD56), and did not react with monoclonal antibodies directed against Fc receptors (CD23/FcεRII, FcεRI) (Strunk et al, submitted for publication).

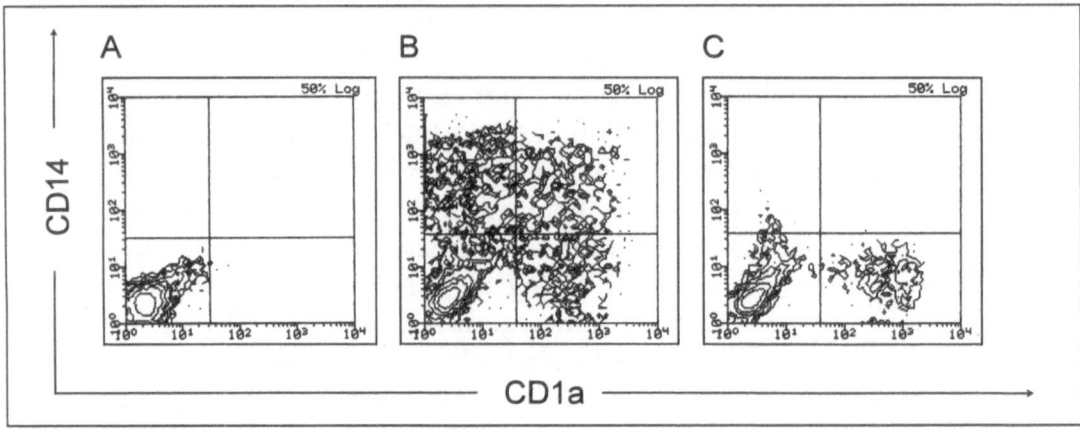

Fig. 2.2. Phenotype of circulating hematopoietic progenitor cells (HPC) and GM-CSF/TNF-α ± IL-4-induced HPC-derived cells. Anti-CD1a (Na1/34-fluorescein isothiocyanate, x-axis) and anti-CD14 (MEM-18-phyco-erythrin, y-axis) immunoreactivity of (A) HPC freshly purified from normal peripheral blood, (B) GM-CSF/ TNF-α-stimulated HPC, and (C) GM-CSF/TNF-α/IL-4-stimulated HPC after two weeks of culture. Results are shown as contour plots as determined with dual-color flow cytometry. (A) HPC circulating in peripheral blood of healthy adults are CD1a⁻/CD14⁻. (B) GM-CSF/TNF-α generates a mixture of CD1a⁺/CD14⁻ cells (lower right quadrant), CD1a⁺/CD14⁺ cells (upper right), CD1a⁻/CD14⁺ cells (upper left), and CD1a⁻/CD14⁻ cells (lower left). (C) Addition of IL-4 to the combination of GM-CSF/TNF-α reduces the overall proliferation and dramatically inhibits the generation of CD14⁺ cells, thus resulting in a relative but not absolute increase in CD1a⁺/CD14⁻ cells (lower right quadrant). Quadrant positions were set after control staining with appropriate isotype control antibodies (mouse IgG2a-fluorescein isothiocyanate vs. mouse IgG1-phycoerythrin). Identical quadrant settings were used for (B) and (C). Cells analyzed in (B) and (C) are derived from the HPC shown in (A) and were cultured under the same conditions except for the presence of IL-4 in addition to GM-CSF/ TNF-α in (C).

Because GM-CSF is known to induce the expression of CD1a, CD1b, and CD1c on monocytes,[28-30] we sought to determine the nature of the in vitro generated CD1a⁺ cells in more detail. Lag reactivity, indicating the presence of BG, was found in 20% of the CD1a⁺ cells. Using transmission electron microscopy, the majority of the CD1a⁺ HPC-derived cells displayed an indented and lobulated nucleus and exhibited numerous short, villous surface projections protruding from the cell membrane. Rod-shaped trilaminar BG were detectable within central portions of the cytoplasm in 10% of the CD1a⁺ cells. A subpopulation of the in vitro generated CD1a⁺ cells can thus be defined as LC.

The CD1a⁺/CD14⁺ cells may belong to the monocyte lineage as evidenced by the IL-4-mediated inhibition of their development. The remaining CD1a⁺/CD14⁻/Lag⁻/BG⁻ cells could be (1) monocytes that have lost CD14 in culture, (2) LC that have already lost or, perhaps, not yet acquired their BG, or (3) represent dendritic cells (Fig. 2.3). The latter hypothesis is supported by data from Romani et al[21] showing that large numbers of CD1a⁺/CD14⁻ immunostimulatory dendritic cells can be generated from a so far unknown precursor in bulk cultures of T cell depleted PBMC with GM-CSF plus IL-4.

The appearance of three distinctive populations of CD1a⁺ cells (CD14⁻/Lag⁺/BG⁺ LC, CD14⁺/Lag⁻/BG⁻ monocytes, and CD14⁻/Lag⁻/BG⁻ dendritic cells) in GM-CSF/TNF-α-stimulated HPC cultures raises questions about the nature of their immediate progenitor cell(s). In the case of the CD1a⁺/CD14⁻/BG⁻ dendritic cells, the results by Romani et al[21] and Sallusto et al[20] indicate that they are derived from a GM-CSF/IL-4-responsive CD34⁻ precursor.

With regard to LC, our finding that incubation of CD14⁺ cells with GM-CSF ± TNF-α ± IL-4, while inducing the expression of CD1 molecules by these cells, never results in the appearance of Lag⁺ cells, argues against a monocyte derivation. Interestingly, CD1a⁺/CD14⁻/BG⁺ LC have so far only been generated in vitro from CD34⁺ cells (Strunk et al, submitted for publication) and CD34⁺ cell-enriched populations.[18] This may indicate that CD34⁺ HPC are the immediate predecessors of LC (Fig. 2.3).

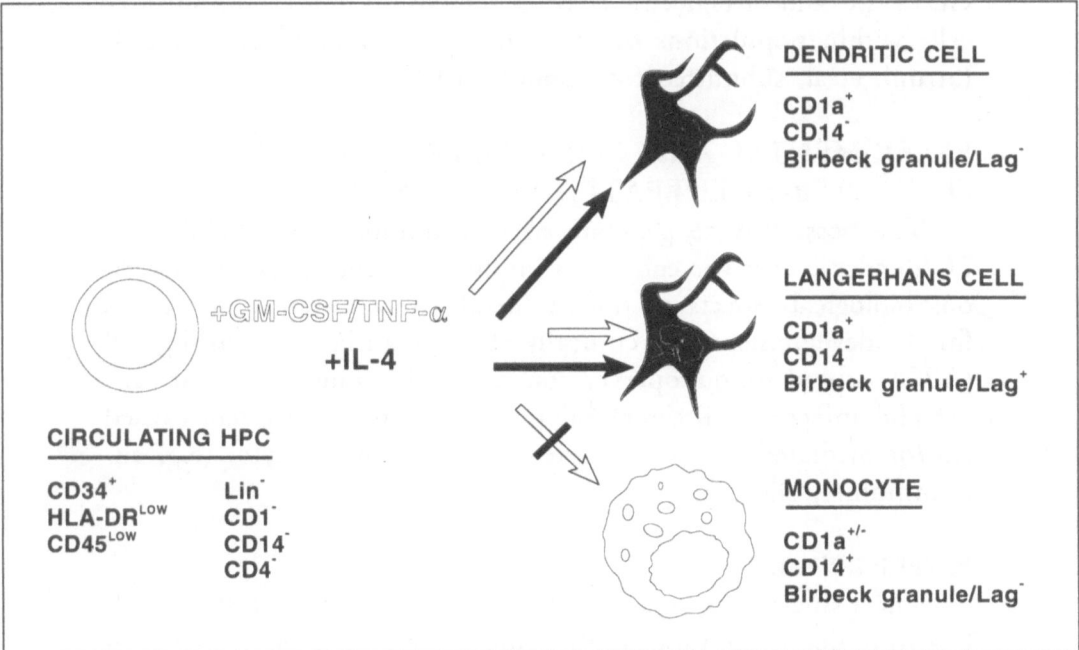

Fig. 2.3. Model for the molecular requirements of CD34⁺ hematopoietic progenitor cells (HPC) for their differentiation and maturation into Langerhans cells, dendritic cells and/or monocytes/macrophages.

To determine whether the in vitro generated CD1a⁺ cells are capable of inducing a primary T cell response, we performed allogeneic mixed leukocyte reactions (MLR). For this purpose, graded numbers of mitomycin C-treated HPC-derived cells were used for the stimulation of 10^5 freshly isolated allogeneic T cells. Repeated experiments showed that in vitro generated HPC-derived cells recovered from GM-CSF/TNF-α ± IL-4-induced cultures elicit a vigorous proliferation of allogeneic T cells, even when used in numbers as low as $3x10^2$. To get further information as to the nature of the principal stimulatory cells in this system, CD1a⁺ cells were removed from the stimulator population. While these CD1a⁻ cells still contained more than 30% HLA-DR⁺ cells, their stimulatory potential was greatly impaired compared to the non CD1a-depleted cell population. This finding is in accordance with the observation by Caux et al[18] that CD1a⁺ but not CD1a⁻ cells generated in vitro with GM-CSF/TNF-α from human cord blood efficiently stimulate allogeneic CD4⁺ T cells.[18] Our further observation that HPC-derived cells generated under conditions which prevent monocyte development, i.e., GM-CSF/TNF-α/IL-4, are as stimulatory as GM-CSF/TNF-α-derived cells, leads us to the conclusion that CD1a⁺ LC and/or dendritic cells are the critical immunostimulatory cells within populations of in vitro generated HPC-derived cells (Strunk et al, submitted for publication).

EXPERIMENTAL AND CLINICAL IMPORTANCE OF IN VITRO GENERATED LANGERHANS CELLS

The possibility to generate sizeable numbers of HPC-derived LC/dendritic cells has enormous implications for the study of various biological aspects of the LC/dendritic cell system as well as for the development of a clinically effective antigen-presenting cell (APC)-assisted immunoprevention and/or immunotherapy of cancer and infectious diseases and perhaps even of disorders caused and/or mediated by abnormal reactions of immunocytes (e.g. autoimmunity, allergy).

EXPERIMENTAL USE

The tissue-culture system described in this chapter should allow us to define the various differentiation and maturation steps that CD34⁺ HPC have to undergo to become a LC/dendritic cell and to study the molecular requirements for the occurrence of these events.

These investigations should also clarify the heavily debated issue concerning the relationship between LC/dendritic cells and cells of the monocyte/macrophage series. Using human skin-grafted SCID/hu mice[31] and/or appropriate organotypic skin equivalents,[32] our method should also be very useful for investigating migratory and homing properties of LC and their immediate and distant precursors and to characterize the molecules involved in these processes.

Simply for reasons of quantity, purity and easy availability, HPC-derived LC/dendritic cells will be an excellent tool (1) to analyze, at a much faster pace than before, the molecular configuration and functional significance of various LC-associated molecules (e.g., cytokines and their receptors, immunoglobulin receptors, costimulatory molecules, adhesins, etc.), (2) to search for new phenotypic and functional features of LC using antibody-based, biochemical, cell biological or molecular biological approaches, (3) to study the molecular mechanisms governing phenotype and function of LC and (4) to test the effects of established and newly developed substances (biological response modifiers, drugs, etc.) on the LC population.

IMMUNOTHERAPY OF CANCER

Although definitive proof is still lacking, there exists substantial evidence that the immune system plays an important role in the prevention and control of cancer. This evidence includes (1) the occasional clinical observation of spontaneous tumor regression, (2) the correlation of this phenomenon with the presence of tumor-infiltrating lymphocytes (TIL), and (3) the in vitro demonstration of the specificity of TIL for the autologous tumor. Due to the weak immunogenicity of, and the occurrence of active immunosuppression by, the cancer, this response often does not successfully combat the neoplasm. As a consequence, numerous attempts have been made to amplify the anti-tumor immune response. These include (1) the direct cytokine-driven expansion of effector cell populations[33] and (2) the vaccination of patients or experimental animals with cancer cells, the immunogenicity of which has been enhanced by the introduction of genes encoding molecules (e.g., cytokines, costimulatory molecules) critically needed for the elicitation of an immune response.[34]

Work from several laboratories indicates that presentation of cancer-associated antigens in the context of professional APC could be a promising alternative approach in cancer immunotherapy. Grabbe et al[35] and Flamand et al[36] have shown that immunization of mice with tumor antigen-pulsed LC/dendritic cells induces a specific resistance against a subsequent inoculation of tumorigenic wild-type cancer cells. Recent in vitro studies by Cohen et al[37] provide direct evidence for the capacity of LC/dendritic cells to process and present tumor-associated antigens to (primed) CD4+ T cells. The presentation of tumor antigens by professional APC is apparently not confined to the MHC class II-restricted pathway[38] but, surprisingly, can also occur in the context of class I molecules.[39] This finding is of great importance because of the requirement for both CD4+ and CD8+ T cells for protective cancer immunity.[34]

Possible strategies for the presentation of cancer-associated antigens by in vitro generated LC/dendritic cells include: (1) LC/dendritic cell pulsing with processing-dependent cancer cell fragments and/or native cancer-associated antigens;[35,36] (2) loading of surface-bound MHC class I or class II molecules with processing-independent tumor antigen-derived peptides;[40] (3) transfection of proliferating LC/dendritic cells with genes encoding for cancer-associated antigens[41] and, finally (4) establishment of highly immunogenic APC/cancer cell chimeras by fusing LC/dendritic cells with the respective tumor cells.[42]

Although the antigen-processing potential of in vitro generated LC has yet to be demonstrated, their derivation from a defined, i.e., not tumor cell-contaminated,[43] precursor cell population (CD34+ HPC) makes them interesting candidates for an APC-based immunotherapy of cancer.

IMMUNOTHERAPY OF INFECTIOUS DISEASES

For a time, it was widely assumed that infectious diseases had been brought under control in at least the industrialized nations. Yet the appearance of the acquired immune deficiency syndrome (AIDS) and the recent resurgence of tuberculosis, including the evolution of multiple drug-resistant strains, show that infectious diseases continue to be major scourges on a worldwide scale and vividly emphasize the need for the development of effective strategies for their treatment and prevention.[44,45] The immune system is an extremely powerful host defense mechanism against microorganisms as evidenced by the success of passive and active vaccination programs against smallpox, tetanus, diphtheria, pertussis, measles, influenza, polio, and hepatitis B. Although the situation is much less satisfactory for other diseases (e.g., mycobacterial diseases, malaria, leishmaniasis, schistosomiasis, human immunodeficiency (HIV) disease), the hope for the development of efficacious vaccines against the microorganisms causing these diseases is based (1) on the increasing knowledge concerning the relative contribution of the various effector mechanisms of the immune system (antibodies, CD4⁺/CD8⁺ T cells and their subpopulations) to the generation of a protective immune response against a given microorganism and (2) a continuously better understanding of the various types of microbial escape mechanisms developing in a particular disease.[45]

Important decisions concerning both the quality and quantity of an immune response occur at the level of the APC, i.e., selection of the appropriate presentation pathway (MHC class I vs. MHC class II) for a given antigen and, as a consequence, selection of the appropriate T cell subset to be activated.[38] In contrast to other APC, LC/dendritic cells have the unique capacity to induce primary and secondary immune responses of all qualities.[7,9,46-48] Given (1) the feasibility of orientating the presentation pathways of selected antigens (e.g., direct delivery of antigens via acid-(in)sensitive liposomes into either the class I or class II presentation pathway[49-51]) and (2) the rapid development of increasingly more effective gene-delivery systems,[34,41,52-54] in vitro generated LC/dendritic cells may serve as ideal vehicles for vaccination. This system is potentially applicable to the disease states listed above but, conceivably, could also be used for the prevention and treatment of virus-induced neoplasms, e.g., Epstein-Barr virus (EBV)-induced diseases (Hodgkin's disease and nasopharyngeal carcinoma),[55] human papillomavirus (HPV)-induced cancer (cervical carcinoma and malignant epithelial proliferation)[56] and perhaps even Kaposi's sarcoma.[57]

TOLERIZATION STRATEGIES

Although LC/dendritic cells are usually viewed and discussed as immunogens for foreign antigens, we should not forget reports demonstrating that ultraviolet (UV) irradiation of LC can modulate their sensitizing potential. Cruz et al[58] reported that intravenous injection of UV-irradiated, hapten-modified LC results in a state of hapten-specific tolerance and Simon et al[59] have shown that LC, upon UV irradiation, lose their capacity to activate T helper (Th) type 1 clones, but retain their stimulatory potential for Th2 clones. Together with the finding that dendritic cells can function as inducers of fetal and neonatal tolerance,[60,61] these observations open the exciting possibility that LC/dendritic cells, upon appropriate phenotypic modulation (e.g., by UV irradiation or other treatment modalities[62]), could be used for silencing auto- and alloreactive as well as allergen-specific T lymphocytes.

REFERENCES

1. Langerhans P. Über die Nerven der menschlichen Haut. Virchows Arch (Pathol Anat) 1868; 44:325-37.

2. Stingl G, Tamaki K, Katz S. Origin and function of epidermal Langerhans cells. Immunol Rev 1980; 53:151-74.

3. Stingl G, Hauser C, Wolff K. The epidermis: An immunologic microenvironment. In: Fitzpatrick TB, Eisen AZ, Wolff K, Freedberg IM, Austen KF, eds. Dermatology in General Medicine. New York: McGraw-Hill, 1993:172-97.

4. Katz SI, Tamaki K, Sachs DH. Epidermal Langerhans cells are derived from cells originating in bone marrow. Nature 1979; 282:324-6.

5. Frelinger JG, Hood L, Hill S et al. Mouse Ia molecules have a bone marrow origin. Nature 1979; 282:321-3.

6. Volc-Platzer B, Stingl G, Wolff K et al. Cytogenetic identification of allogeneic epidermal Langerhans cells in a bone-marrow-graft recipient. N Engl J Med 1984; 310:1123-4.

7. Stingl G, Shevach E. Langerhans cells as antigen-presenting cells. In: Schuler G, ed. Epidermal Langerhans Cells. Boca Raton: CRC Press, 1991:159-90.

8. Bos JD, Kapsenberg ML. The skin immune system: progress in cutaneous biology. Immunol Today 1993; 14:75-8.

9. Steinman RM, Witmer-Pack M, Inaba K. Dendritic cells: Antigen presentation, accessory function and clinical relevance. In: Kamperdijk EWA, Nieuwenhuis P, Hoefsmit ECM, eds. Dendritic Cells in Fundamental and Clinical Immunology. New York: Plenum Press, 1994:1-9.

10. Klinkert WEF. Rat bone marrow precursors develop into dendritic accessory cells under the influence of conditioned medium. Immunobiol 1984; 168:414-24.

11. Bowers WE, Berkowitz MR. Differentiation of dendritic cells in cultures of rat bone marrow cells. J Exp Med 1986; 163:872-83.

12. Reid CDL, Fryer PR, Clifford C et al. Identification of hematopoietic progenitors of macrophages and dendritic Langerhans cells (DL-CFU) in human bone marrow and peripheral blood. Blood 1990; 76:1139-49.

13. Inaba K, Inaba M, Romani N et al. Generation of large numbers of dendritic cells from mouse bone marrow cultures supplemented with granulocyte/macrophage colony-stimulating factor. J Exp Med 1992; 176:1693-1702.

14. Inaba K, Inaba M, Deguchi M et al. Granulocytes, macrophages, and dendritic cells arise from a common major histocompatibility complex class II-negative progenitor in mouse bone marrow. Proc Natl Acad Sci USA 1993; 90:3038-42.

15. Scheicher C, Mehlig M, Zecher R et al. Dendritic cells from mouse bone marrow: in vitro differentiation using low doses of recombinant granulocyte-macrophage colony-stimulating factor. J Immunol Meth 1992; 154:253-64.

16. Reid CDL, Stackpole A, Meager A et al. Interactions of tumor necrosis factor with granulocyte-macrophage colony-stimulating factor and other cytokines in the regulation of dendritic cell growth in vitro from early bipotent CD34+ progenitors in human bone marrow. J Immunol 1992; 149:2681-8.

17. Santiago-Schwarz F, Belilos E, Diamond B et al. TNF in combination with GM-CSF enhances the differentiation of neonatal cord blood stem cells into dendritic cells and macrophages. J Leukoc Biol 1992; 52:274-81.

18. Caux C, Dezutter-Dambuyant C, Schmitt D et al. GM-CSF and TNF-α cooperate in the generation of dendritic Langerhans cells. Nature 1992; 360:258-61.

19. Inaba K, Steinman RM, Witmer-Pack MD et al. Identification of proliferating dendritic cell precursors in mouse blood. J Exp Med 1992; 175:1157-67.

20. Sallusto F, Lanzavecchia A. Efficient presentation of soluble antigen by cultured dendritic cells is maintained by granulocyte/macrophage colony-stimulating factor plus interleukin 4 and downregulated by tumor necrosis factor α. J Exp Med 1994; 179: 1109-18.

21. Romani N, Gruner S, Brang D et al. Proliferating dendritic cell progenitors in human blood. J Exp Med 1994; 180:83-93.

22. Gabbianelli M, Sargiacomo M, Pelosi E et al. "Pure" human hematopoietic progenitors: Permissive action of basic fibroblast growth factor. Science 1990; 249:1561-4.

23. Bender JG, Unverzagt KL, Walker DE et al. Identification and comparison of CD34-positive cells and their subpopulations from normal peripheral blood and bone marrow using multicolor flow cytometry. Blood 1991; 77:2591-6.

24. Kato K, Radbruch A. Isolation and characterization of CD34+ hematopoietic stem cells from human peripheral blood by high-gradient magnetic cell sorting. Cytometry 1993; 14:384-92.

25. Picker LJ, Michie SA, Rott LS et al. A unique phenotype of skin-associated lymphocytes in humans. Am J Pathol 1990; 136:1053-68.

26. Koszik F, Strunk D, Simonitsch I et al. Expression of monoclonal antibody HECA-452-defined E-selectin ligands on Langerhans cells

in normal and diseased skin. J Invest Dermatol 1994; 102:773-80.

27. Jansen JH, Wientjens G-JHM, Fibbe WE et al. Inhibition of human macrophage colony formation by interleukin 4. J Exp Med 1989; 170:577-82.

28. Rossi G, Heveker N, Thiele B et al. Development of a Langerhans cell phenotype from peripheral blood monocytes. Immunol Letters 1992; 31:189-98.

29. Porcelli S, Morita CT, Brenner MB. CD1b restricts the response of human CD4⁻8⁻ T lymphocytes to a microbial antigen. Nature 1992; 360:593-7.

30. Kasinrerk W, Baumruker T, Majdic O et al. CD1 molecule expression on human monocytes induced by granulocyte-macrophage colony-stimulating factor. J Immunol 1993; 150:579-84.

31. Murray AG, Petzelbauer P, Hughes CCW et al. Human T-cell-mediated destruction of allogeneic dermal microvessels in a severe combined immunodeficient mouse. Proc Natl Acad Sci USA 1994; 91:9146-50.

32. Coulomb B, Lebreton C, Dubertret L. The skin equivalent: A model for skin and general pharmacology. In: Maibach HI, Lowe NJ, eds. Models in Dermatol. Basel: Karger, 1989:20-9.

33. Rosenberg SA. Gene therapy of cancer. In: De Vita, Hellman S, Rosenberg SA, eds. Important Advances in Oncology. Philadelphia: J.B. Lippincott, 1992:17-38.

34. Pardoll D. Cancer vaccines. Immunol Today 1993; 14:310-6.

35. Grabbe S, Bruvers S, Gallo RS et al. Tumor antigen presentation by murine epidermal cells. J Immunol 1991; 146:3656-61.

36. Flamand V, Sornasse T, Thielemans K et al. Murine dendritic cells pulsed *in vitro* with tumor antigen induce tumor resistance *in vivo*. Eur J Immunol 1994; 24:605-10.

37. Cohen PJ, Cohen PA, Rosenberg SA et al. Murine epidermal Langerhans cells and splenic dendritic cells present tumor-associated antigens to primed T cells. Eur J Immunol 1994; 24:315-9.

38. Germain RN, Margulies DH. The biochemistry and cell biology of antigen processing and presentation. Annu Rev Immunol 1993; 11:403-50.

39. Huang AYC, Golumbek P, Ahmadzadeh M et al. Role of bone marrow-derived cells in presenting MHC class I-restricted tumor antigens. Science 1994; 264:961-5.

40. Slingluff CL, Hunt DF, Engelhard VH. Direct analysis of tumor-associated peptide antigens. Curr Opin Immunol 1994; 6:733-40.

41. Boon T, Cerottini J-C, Van den Eynde B et al. Tumor antigens recognized by T lymphocytes. Annu Rev Immunol 1994; 12:337-65.

42. Guo Y, Wu M, Chen H et al. Effective tumor vaccine generated by fusion of hepatoma cells with activated B cells. Science 1994; 263:518-20.

43. Schlimok G, Pantel K, Lindemann F et al. Model for measurement of micrometastasis in epithelial tumors. In: van Furth R, ed.

Hemopoietic growth factors and mononuclear phagocytes. Basel: Karger, 1993:168-76.

44. Paul WE. Infectious diseases and the immune system. Scientific American, The Immune System 1993; 57:57-63.

45. Lambert PH. New vaccines for the world-needs and prospects. The Immunologist 1993; 1:50-5.

46. Inaba K, Steinman R. Protein-specific helper T-lymphocyte formation initiated by dendritic cells. Science 1985; 229:475-9.

47. Inaba K, Young JW, Steinman RM. Direct activation of CD8⁺ cytotoxic T lymphocytes by dendritic cells. J Exp Med 1987; 166:182-90.

48. Elbe A, Schleischitz S, Strunk D et al. Fetal skin-derived MHC class I⁺, MHC class II⁻ dendritic cells stimulate MHC class I-restricted responses of unprimed CD8⁺ T cells. J Immunol 1994; 153:2878-89.

49. Harding CV, Collins DS, Kanagawa O et al. Liposome-encapsuled antigens engender lysosomal processing for class II MHC presentation and cytosolic processing for class I presentation. J Immunol 1991; 147:2860-3.

50. Noguchi Y, Noguchi T, Sato T et al. Priming for in vitro and in vivo anti-human T lymphotropic virus type 1 cellular immunity by virus-related protein reconstituted into liposome. J Immunol 1991; 146:3599-3603.

51. Alving CR, Wassef NM. Novel vaccines and adjuvants: Mechanisms of action. AIDS Res Hum Retroviruses 1994; 10:S91-6.

52. Zatloukal K, Wagner E, Cotten M et al. Transferinfection: A highly efficient way to express gene constructs in eucaryotic cells. Ann NY Acad Sci 1992; 660:136-53.

53. Kerr WG, Mulé JJ. Gene therapy: Current status and future prospects. J Leukoc Biol 1994; 56:210-4.

54. Wang B, Merva M, Dang K et al. Vectors and novel vaccines. AIDS Res Hum Retroviruses 1994; 10:S35-44.

55. Chopra R, Goldstone AH. Recent advances in Hodgkin's disease. Curr Opin Hematol 1994; 1:285-94.

56. Wu T. Immunology of the human papilloma virus in relation to cancer. Curr Opin Immunol 1994; 6:746-54.

57. Chang Y, Cesarman E, Pessin MS et al. Identification of herpes virus-like DNA sequences in AIDS-associated Kaposi's sarcoma. Science 1994; 266:1865-9.

58. Cruz Jr PD, Nixon-Fulton J, Tigelaar RE et al. Disparate effects of in vitro low-dose UVB irradiation on intravenous immunization with purified epidermal cell subpopulations for the induction of contact hypersensitivity. J Invest Dermatol 1989; 92:160-5.

59. Simon JC, Tigelaar RE, Bergstresser PR et al. Ultraviolet B radiation converts Langerhans cells from immunogenic to tolerogenic antigen-presenting cells. Induction of specific clonal anergy in CD4⁺ T helper 1 cells. J Immunol 1991; 146:486-91.

60. Matzinger P, Guerder S. Does T-cell tolerance require a dedicated antigen-presenting cell? Nature 1989; 338:74-6.
61. Inaba M, Inaba K, Hosono M et al. Distinct mechanisms of neonatal tolerance induced by dendritic cells and thymic B cells. J Exp Med 1991; 173:549-56.
62. Gruner S, Diezel W, Strunk D et al. Inhibition of Langerhans cell ATPase and contact sensitization by lanthanide's-Role of T-suppressor cells. J Invest Dermatol 1991; 97:478-85.

CHAPTER 3

CYTOKINE RECEPTORS ON EPIDERMAL LANGERHANS CELLS

Eckhart Kämpgen, Nikolaus Romani, Franz Koch,
Andreas Eggert, Gerold Schuler

INTRODUCTION

Epidermal Langerhans cells (LC) are considered members of the dendritic cell system which constitutes a distinct lineage of major histocompatibility complex (MHC) class II-expressing leukocytes specialized to initiate primary immune responses.[1] Work of recent years has established LC as a beautiful model to study the life history of dendritic cells and has greatly augmented the current concept that immunostimulatory lymphoid dendritic cells originate from immature nonlymphoid precursor cells in peripheral tissues.[2] Accordingly immature "tissue dendritic cells," such as LC in situ, capture and process antigen in the periphery. They then shut off further processing and, while maturation into potent immunostimulatory "lymphoid dendritic cells" takes place, migrate to the draining lymphoid organs where the immunogen has maximal chance to encounter specific T cells.[3] Immature "tissue dendritic cells" in other organs such as lung or liver have now been characterized. However, the functional properties of dendritic cells in their different maturational stages and the corresponding cellular and molecular mechanisms have so far been best analyzed with epidermal LC as a model.

The Immune Functions of Epidermal Langerhans Cells, edited by Heidrun Moll.
© 1995 R.G. Landes Company.

When freshly isolated, immature LC are weak stimulators of primary T cell responses.[4] They are, however, extremely efficient in processing exogenous protein antigens and presenting them as immunogenic MHC class II–peptide complexes to primed T cells.[5] This remarkable capacity correlates with the presence of many acidic organelles within freshly isolated LC and a very high rate of MHC class II and invariant chain synthesis.[6,7] Upon short-term culture (2 to 3 days), LC change morphologically and phenotypically, and their functions are expressed in a reciprocal fashion: Cultured LC become powerful stimulators of resting T cells, reflected now by the capacity to bind (cluster) resting T cells in an antigen-independent fashion.[8] At the same time, cultured LC lose their antigen-processing skills, i.e., they completely shut off MHC class II synthesis and certain acidic organelles are lost. A very distinctive feature of maturating LC, as opposed to macrophages, is that the newly synthesized class II–peptide complexes remain stably on the cell surface, enabling LC to retain immunogen until arrival in the lymphoid organ and to sensitize T cells to the antigens they have encountered in the periphery.[7] In all respects, cultured LC now resemble lymphoid dendritic cells and hence LC in situ may be regarded as immature "tissue dendritic cells" which upon appropriate stimuli mature into classical lymphoid dendritic cells.[3]

It is obvious that such dynamic cell functions of maturation and migration need to be tightly regulated, and cytokines appear to be crucial in this regulation. Here we will briefly review current knowledge on responses of LC to cytokines and will then discuss data from our laboratory concerning the expression of certain cytokine receptors by LC in different maturational stages. Based on these data, a hypothetical model of early events within the epidermis leading to the onset of maturation and migration will be proposed.

CYTOKINES AFFECTING EPIDERMAL LANGERHANS CELLS

Langerhans cells constitute only a minor subpopulation (1-3%) of all epidermal cells, the most being keratinocytes, which have been recognized as a potent source of numerous cytokines. Therefore, in vitro cytokine effects on LC can only be analyzed using highly purified LC populations. Such studies became feasible when positive selection by fluorescence-activated cell sorter (FACS) or panning techniques are allowed to reproducibly enrich LC at the required purity.[9] Recently, cytokines directly acting on and influencing LC have been identified.

IN VITRO RESPONSES OF LANGERHANS CELLS TO CYTOKINES

Whereas resident LC in the epidermis are relatively long-lived, freshly isolated and highly enriched (i.e., keratinocyte-depleted) LC rapidly die when cultured in plain serum-containing medium. If, however, LC are poorly enriched (less than 60%), or keratinocyte-conditioned medium is added to the culture, most LC survive for a three-day period and undergo a series of phenotypical and functional alterations: LC develop numerous sheet-like extensions, the capacity to process native antigen is lost and so are certain macrophage markers, the surface expression of MHC class II antigens is upregulated and a very potent stimulatory capacity for resting T cells develops. In vitro studies using highly enriched LC led to the discovery of granulocyte/macrophage colony-stimulating factor (GM-CSF) as the keratinocyte-derived cytokine responsible for this maturational process.[10,11] If purified LC are cultured with recombinant GM-CSF, there is a 10- to 30-fold increase in the sensitizing function of LC for resting T cells, which is enhanced another twofold by further addition of interleukin (IL) 1α or IL-1β.[11] IL-1 alone, however, does not sustain LC viability. There is evidence that the sensitizing function-promoting effects of GM-CSF and IL-1 are mediated by an increased capacity of LC to bind resting T cells in an antigen-independent fashion, possibly by upregulating the expression of a yet unknown critical adhesion molecule (cluster molecule). This clustering capacity, allowing specific T cell receptors to interact with immunogen (peptide–MHC complex), is currently regarded as an essential prerequisite for the initiation of primary immune responses.[12] In addition, GM-CSF has been shown to induce LC and dendritic cells to upregulate their surface expression of costimulatory signals such as B7-1 and B7-2,[13] which are critical for stimulation of resting T cells and T helper cells of type 1 (Th1).

Tumor necrosis factor α (TNF-α), a second mediator capable of maintaining the survival of murine LC in vitro was recently identified.[14] If purified LC are cultured with recombinant TNF-α, similar morphological and phenotypical changes including upregulation of MHC class II molecules can be observed. In con-

trast to GM-CSF-treated LC, however, LC cultured with TNF-α
remain poor stimulators of resting T cells. We have some evidence
that impaired clustering capacity of TNF-LC might account for
this difference.[15] As is the case with GM-CSF, LC downregulate
their antigen processing capacity upon culture with TNF-α. However, they also progressively lose immunogenic peptides from their
MHC class II molecules during the culture period.[16] Thus, TNF-α
interrupts the antigen-presenting function of epidermal LC, possibly due to an increased turnover of MHC class II-peptide complexes (F. Koch, E. Kämpgen, N. Koch et al, manuscript in preparation). In addition, purified TNF-α-cultured LC were recently
shown to induce antigen-specific tolerance in Th1 clones. This
capacity to induce clonal anergy was reflected by a selective deficiency in expression of the costimulatory molecule B7-1
(E. Kämpgen, F. Koch, A. Enk et al, manuscript in preparation).
A comparable tolerizing capacity of LC on Th1 clones has already
been described as an effect of IL-10 (see chapter 4 by Enk and
Katz). However, IL-10 *per se* does not sustain viability of LC and,
in contrast to TNF-α, induces LC to become tolerizing antigen-
presenting cells (APC) even in the presence of GM-CSF.[17]

   None of several other available cytokines tested so far including macrophage-CSF (M-CSF) and granulocyte-CSF (G-CSF) exert a viability-sustaining effect on LC. However, combinations of
certain cytokines, which have not yet been analyzed in detail, might
influence the viability of LC or alter functional capacities. Specifically, we do not know how upregulation of MHC class II, which
occurs even if LC are placed in plain medium, and expression of a
series of adhesion molecules are induced and controlled during culture. In this respect, other mediators of inflammation like pros-
taglandins or leukotrienes should also be taken into account.[18]

IN VIVO RESPONSES OF LANGERHANS CELLS TO CYTOKINES

   Whereas in vitro experiments identified GM-CSF and IL-1 as
critical mediators of LC maturation and point to a downregulatory
role for TNF-α in antigen presentation, in vivo data on cytokine
effects are still sparse and mainly indirect. Attempts to induce in
vivo LC maturation and migration in mouse skin by local as well
as systemic injections of high doses of GM-CSF did not alter LC
density[19] or phenotype (F. Koch, unpublished results) within the
epidermis, suggesting that LC in situ are not responsive to GM-CSF

without additional stimuli. Yet, painting mouse skin with contact sensitizers results in a 30-40% decrease in LC density after 24 hours, probably reflecting the onset of LC migration to regional lymph nodes. This effect is not seen using nonsensitizers or tolerogen. In a recent study by Enk[20] (and see chapter 4 by Enk and Katz) the cytokine-production profile of epidermal cells in the induction phase of contact sensitivity was analyzed. Whereas GM-CSF and TNF-α mRNA was uniformly upregulated by epidermal cells in response to haptens as well as irritants, mRNA for IL-1α and IL-1β, interferon (IFN)-induced protein 10 (IP-10) and macrophage-inflammatory protein 2 (MIP-2) increased only if contact sensitizers were applied. Interestingly, LC themselves could be identified as a source of the IL-1β production within the epidermis.[21] These results may indicate that one or all of these cytokines are involved in events that make LC emigrate from the epidermis.

Some in vivo experiments add to a potential immunosuppressive role for TNF-α. Thus, after intradermal injection of TNF-α there is a marked inhibition of subsequent contact sensitization.[22] TNF-α was also shown to impede the development of immunity that could otherwise be induced by injecting in vitro pulsed epidermal LC into syngenic recipients.[23] On the other hand, some in vivo data point to a role for TNF-α as a stimulus to LC emigration from the epidermis. Intradermal injections of TNF-α but not GM-CSF led to a decrease in LC density and an increase in dendritic cell numbers in the draining lymph nodes.[24]

In addition, putative immunosuppressive effects on epidermal LC have been described for IL-10 in vivo (see chapter 4 by Enk and Katz). Dermal injection of IL-10 before allergen treatment inhibited the induction of a contact-hypersensitivity reaction and induced antigen-specific tolerance. This effect of IL-10 was attributed to inhibition of proinflammatory cytokines within the skin.[25]

None of these experiments, however, can be regarded as a proof that a given cytokine really does influence LC and not exert its function via induction of other cytokines. In any case, in situ LC are exposed to a mixture of different cytokines and a fine-tuned balance of these might govern the outcome after antigenic challenge of the skin. To better understand which of the cytokines invoked may directly act on LC, we set out to determine the expression and the expression kinetics of specific cytokine receptors on murine epidermal LC in different maturational stages, i.e., on freshly prepared "immature" versus cultured "mature" LC/lymphoid dendritic cells.

CYTOKINE RECEPTORS
ON EPIDERMAL LANGERHANS CELLS

For several reasons, data on cytokine receptors expressed by LC have been difficult to obtain and hence are very sparse. First, cell-surface expression of cytokine receptors is generally very low (a few hundred to thousand receptors per cell), making immuno-labeling attempts difficult or impossible. Second, the classical method of receptor quantification, which is to measure the binding of a radiolabeled ligand to a defined cell population in the presence or absence of excessive unlabeled ligand, usually requires many cells to compensate for the low receptor numbers (at least 10^6 cells per datapoint). Radioligand binding assays thus could not be applied until the recent development of a modified panning technique[9] that enabled us to obtain good yields of highly enriched LC from freshly prepared as well as cultured epidermal cells. Third, cytokine receptor molecules are often trypsin sensitive. Since two trypsinization steps are required for the purification of freshly isolated LC, such binding assays cannot be applied to analyze trypsin sensitive receptors on freshly prepared LC. Finally, the benefit of molecular biology studies critically depends on the availability of mRNA from virtually 100% pure LC populations. Therefore, despite an increasing number of cDNA probes and polymerase chain reaction (PCR) primers, hard data are still lacking. In spite of these obstacles, some informative data on LC expression of cytokine receptors have been procured recently.[26]

GM-CSF RECEPTORS

Freshly isolated LC are highly responsive to GM-CSF. Since GM-CSF receptors are trypsin-sensitive they cannot be quantified on fresh LC by classical binding assays as outlined above. We therefore used highly purified cultured LC (from three-day epidermal cell cultures) and mature spleen dendritic cells. Equilibrium binding studies with ^{125}I-labeled recombinant murine GM-CSF (see Table 3.1) revealed surprisingly high numbers of high-affinity receptors for GM-CSF on cultured LC (approx. 3×10^3 per cell) and dendritic cells (approx. 2×10^3 per cell) as compared to macro-

Table 3.1. Binding characteristics of recombinant murine ^{125}I-GM-CSF to purified murine cultured LC, spleen dendritic cells and J774 cells*

Cell type	GM-CSF receptors (number/cell ± SD)	K_d (pM)
three-day cultured LC	3,248 (±168)	745 (±198)
spleen dendritic cells	2,644 (±174)	544 (± 65)
1774 macrophage line	858 (± 41)	1170 (±244)

* Adapted with permission from Kämpgen E, Koch F, Heufler C et al. J Exp Med 1994; 179:1767-76.

phage standard cell lines (<1 x 10³ per cell). Comparable data were obtained using either BALB/c or C3H mice. Thus far such amounts of GM-CSF receptors had only been detected on granulocyte/macrophage progenitor cells.[27] Data from Scatchard plot analysis were compatible with a single class of GM-CSF receptors with a dissociation constant (K_d) of 500-1000 pM being expressed by both cultured LC and dendritic cells.

The high-affinity GM-CSF receptor has been shown to consist of two subunits: A low-affinity α chain (Cdw116) specifically binds GM-CSF, but is unable to transduce signals. A second, β, chain converts the low-affinity receptor (K_d >10,000 pM) to high affinity (K_d <50 pM).[28] This β chain, also common to IL-3 and IL-5 receptors, transduces signals but is unable to bind ligand.[29] Interestingly, overexpression of the β chain in relation to the α chain resulted in generation of intermediate-affinity GM-CSF receptors with a K_d of 300-700.[30] Maximal biological activity of GM-CSF is often seen at concentrations many fold less than the K_d of its receptor, when only a subset of receptors is occupied.[31] The observation that about 60 pM of GM-CSF are sufficient to maintain viability of LC and dendritic cells in vitro is therefore compatible with the expression of a single class of intermediate-affinity GM-CSF receptors on LC and dendritic cells. However, due to methodical constraints when dealing with trace populations such as dendritic cells and LC, expression of small numbers of additional GM-CSF receptors with lower or higher K_d cannot be excluded.

Deduced from in vivo studies (see above), epidermal LC in situ most likely do not express functional GM-CSF receptors. Our findings of high numbers of a single class of intermediate-affinity GM-CSF receptors on functionally mature spleen dendritic cells and cultured LC thus suggest strong upregulation of the β-subunit of the GM-CSF receptor during maturation of immature precursors such as freshly isolated LC into fully mature dendritic cells. IL-1 and TNF-α have recently been shown to induce selective upregulation of the β-subunit of the GM-CSF receptor in hemopoietic cells.[32] Hence, both are likely to be involved in the upregulation of GM-CSF receptors as a key event in LC maturation.

M-CSF RECEPTORS

Hitherto M-CSF has not been shown to exert any effect on murine LC or dendritic cells. In accordance, we did not find receptors for M-CSF on cultured LC and spleen dendritic cells as determined by radioligand-binding assays with ^{125}I-labeled recombinant human M-CSF.[26] Interestingly, expression of mRNA for c-fms, which is a homologue to the receptor for M-CSF, was found in freshly prepared murine and also resident human LC.[33] A better enrichment technique has now enabled us to readdress this issue with highly purified fresh LC. Cells were cultured for 12 hours in plain medium to allow for re-expression of the trypsin sensitive M-CSF receptors, then radioligand-binding assays were performed. These experiments procured evidence that 12 hour-cultured LC do express specific receptors for M-CSF and thus confirm the aforementioned molecular biology data (manuscript in preparation). However, LC and dendritic cells do develop normally in mice deficient for M-CSF.[34] Thus, M-CSF receptors on LC presumably are nonfunctional and, furthermore, downregulated during maturation.

TNF RECEPTORS AND IL-10 RECEPTORS

Hitherto no definite data on the expression of receptors for TNF and IL-10 by dendritic cells have been procured. However, the in vitro effects of TNF-α on the viability and functional capacities of highly enriched epidermal LC strongly imply the expression of functional TNF-receptors on freshly obtained LC.[14] Furthermore, TNF-α cooperates with GM-CSF in the generation of dendritic cells[35] and LC[36] from progenitor cells in bone marrow or blood, possibly via upregulation of GM-CSF receptors.[37] There are two receptors for TNF: a 55-kD type I receptor (CD120a), expressed, e.g., by keratinocytes;[38] and a 75-kD type II receptor (CD120b) which is more restricted to hematopoietic cells.[39] Both receptors are functionally competent and bind TNF-α and TNF-β (lymphotoxin); however the mouse type II receptor does not bind human TNF-α. Based on our finding that viability of murine LC can be maintained by human TNF-β (unpublished data) but not human TNF-α,[14] epidermal LC likely express p75-type II TNF receptors. In accordance with this presumption are recent data on prevention of apoptotic cell death in LC and dendritic cell populations by TNF-α,[40] whereas in contrast the p55 receptor has been implicated in the opposite, i.e., induction of programmed cell death.[41]

In vivo data on cytokines affecting epidermal LC viability and function usually are not conclusive as to whether these cytokines directly influence LC via specific receptors or indirectly via induction or suppression of cytokine production by epidermal keratinocytes and other dermal cells. This holds true especially for TNF-α, known to exert several effects on keratinocytes, e.g., induction of IL-1α and IL-1 receptor antagonist,[42] but also for IL-10, shown to inhibit cytokine production by keratinocytes (IL-1α and TNF-α) and presumably also by epidermal LC (IL-1β).[25]

Despite several in vitro studies dealing with IL-10 effects on dendritic cells and LC, there is still no clear-cut evidence for the expression of IL-10 receptors on LC dendritic cells. Hitherto studies were performed either with less enriched LC/dendritic cell populations,[17] or in the presence of T cells,[43] or with purified LC of low viability that had been cultured with IL-10 for extended times in the absence of viability-sustaining cytokines.[44] Thus, conclusive data on the expression of high-affinity IL-10 receptors (K_d <100 pM) in LC and dendritic cell populations are badly needed.

IL-2 Receptors

The high-affinity IL-2 receptor (K_d <20 pM) is a heterotrimer consisting of an α, β and γ chain.[45] Whereas the α chain (CD25) and β chain (CD122) both bind IL-2 with low affinity (K_d >50 μM), no ligand is bound by the γ chain, which constitutes the common functional component of the IL-4, IL-7, IL-15 and likely also the IL-9 and IL-13 receptors. Intermediate-affinity (K_d <1 μM) IL-2 receptor complexes are formed from α/γ or β/γ heterodimers.

Expression of the IL-2 receptor α chain (CD25) has been demonstrated by FACS analysis on cultured human[46] and murine[47] epidermal LC, rat lymph-borne veiled dendritic cells in culture with GM-CSF[48] and dendritic cells generated from precursor cells in mouse blood.[49] In addition, small amounts of CD25 were detected on murine spleen and thymic dendritic cells.[50] However, by cytofluorometry we could not detect IL-2 receptor β-chain (CD122) expression on either lymphoid dendritic cells or on freshly isolated or cultured murine and rat LC (E. Loncarek, J. Hehn, P. Keikavoussi et al, manuscript in preparation; monoclonal antibodies to rat CD122 were kindly supplied by T. Hünig, Würzburg). Whereas CD122 expression could not be detected on human LC either, expression of γ chain-specific mRNA was recently found in purified human LC by PCR (personal communication by T. Bieber, Munich). In addition, T. Bieber has obtained first evidence for a functional role of IL-2 on LC, in that IL-2 might be involved in homing of LC to T cell areas of lymphoid organs. These fascinating new data might also point to a new signaling cascade of the IL-2 receptor in LC, since IL-2 receptor signaling normally requires heterodimerization of the cytoplasmic domains of both the β and γ chains.[51]

IL-1 RECEPTORS

There are two distantly related proteins, IL-1α and IL-1β, that possess all of the biological activities previously ascribed to IL-1.[52] Both are synthesized as intracytoplasmic precursor proteins and processed prior to release from the cells. In contrast to pro-IL-1α, pro-IL-1β is a nonfunctional protein and processed by a specific IL-1β-converting enzyme (ICE) which is not found in keratinocytes.[53] Many cells that secrete IL-1 also produce an IL-1 receptor antagonist protein (IL-1Ra) showing structural relation to IL-1β.[54] In addition, an intracellular IL-1Ra (icIL-1Ra) lacking a substantial portion of the hydrophobic leader sequence has recently been identified in keratinocytes.[55] IL-1 receptors also exist in two types, which both bind to overlapping sites on IL-1α and IL-1β.[56] The 80-kD type I receptor (Cdw121a) binds IL-1α, IL-1β, pro-IL-1α and the IL-1Ra with a similar K_d of <100 pM and is the principal mediator of all IL-1 responses.[57] The smaller type II IL-1 receptor of 60 kD (CDw121b) cannot transmit IL-1 signals and, since it binds IL-1α and IL-1Ra with 10 to 100-fold lower affinity, may be regarded as a relatively specific antagonist for IL-1β.[58] The IL-1Ra is an antagonist for both IL-1α and IL-1β, because it binds irreversibly to the signaling type I receptor. Furthermore, substantial amounts of soluble type II receptors and smaller amounts of type I receptors can be detected in body fluids as well as in supernatants of cell lines that express IL-1 receptors.[59] Taken together, real IL-1 should be regarded as a mixture of agonist components (pro-IL-1α, IL-1α and IL-1β) and antagonists (IL-1Ra, icIL-1Ra, IL-1 receptor type II and soluble IL-1 receptors type I and II), which modulate the specific biological activities of the agonists. Therefore, the extent of biological responses to IL-1 will be determined mainly by the expression of functional type I IL-1 receptors on the target cells.

Our interest in IL-1 receptors on LC/dendritic cells was stimulated by the finding that IL-1 could enhance the immunostimulatory function of epidermal LC[11] as well as lymphoid dendritic cells.[60] Furthermore, IL-1 is a candidate cytokine involved in upregulation of GM-CSF receptors on epidermal LC in situ following skin treatment with contact sensitizers.[32] Because of the trypsin sensitivity of IL-1 receptors we first used purified spleen dendritic cells and mature three-day cultured LC and performed classical radioligand binding studies. Using human recombinant ^{125}I-IL-1α (see Table 3.2), we detected about 500 IL-1 receptors on cultured LC and 70 receptors on spleen dendritic cells.[26] One pilot experiment with one-day cultured LC, of the utmost difficulty to procure in sufficient numbers, revealed about 1200 IL-1 receptors per cell. This is the first evidence that immature LC might express high numbers of IL-1 receptors which are downregulated upon maturation. Scatchard-plot analysis of the binding data was compatible with a single class of high-affinity binding sites (K_d of <100 pM) on both LC and dendritic cells (see Table 3.2). The presence of type I IL-1 receptors on LC and dendritic cells was further strengthened by showing that ^{125}I-IL-1α binding to LC and dendritic cells could (1) be competed against effectively for by human IL-1Ra, which does not bind to type II IL-1 receptors, and (2) be completely inhibited by monoclonal antibodies to murine type I IL-1 receptors. In addition, affinity cross-linking of ^{125}I-IL-1β to IL-1 receptors on LC and dendritic cells resulted in complexes of about 100 kD (80 kD type I receptor plus bound IL-1β of 18 kD) that were also found on EL4-NOB1 control cells known to express high numbers of type I IL-1 receptors. As can be seen in Figure 3.1, affinity-crosslinking of IL-1 receptors on one-day cultured LC produced a more intense band compared to that seen

Table 3.2. Binding characteristics of recombinant human ^{125}I-IL-1α to purified murine one-day and three-day cultured LC, spleen dendritic cells and EL4 control cells*

Cell type	IL-1 receptors (number/cell SD)	K_d (pM)
one-day cultured LC	~ 1,200	
three-day cultured LC	490 (± 20)	58 (± 5) spleen
dendritic cells	69 (± 11)	85 (±22)
EL4-NOB1	2,150 (± 40)	61 (± 4)

* Adapted with permission from Kämpgen E, Koch F, Heufler C et al. J Exp Med 1994; 179:1767-76.

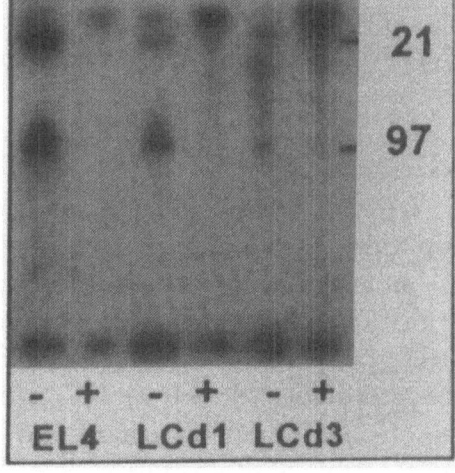

Fig. 3.1. Characterization of IL-1 receptors on epidermal Langerhans cells by affinity cross-linking. 2 x 10⁶ purified epidermal LC from BALB/c mice cultured for one day (LCd1) and three days (LCd3) and 5 x 10⁶ EL4-NOB1 cells (expressing the murine type I IL-1 receptor) were cross-linked to recombinant human ^{125}I-IL-1β in the absence (-) or presence (+) of a 50-fold molar excess of unlabeled IL-1β. Cell extracts were analyzed by sodium dodecyl sulfate-polyacrylamide gel electrophoresis (SDS-PAGE) on a 10-15% gradient gel. Adapted with permission from Kämpgen E, Koch F, Heufler C et al. J Exp Med 1994; 179:1767-76.

with mature three-day cultured LC, both migrating at 97 kD as did the type I IL-1 receptor complexes obtained from EL4 cells.

Further evidence that immature LC express large numbers of IL-1 receptors came from cytofluorography studies. When epidermal cells were prepared using very low trypsin concentrations, MHC class II-positive LC could all be nicely stained with three different mAbs to the murine type I IL-1 receptor (M15 and M5 obtained from S. Dower[61] and 1593-01 obtained from Genzyme), as could be EL-4 control cells. Since we were unable to stain one-day cultured LC, three-day cultured LC or dendritic cells with these mAbs, downregulation of IL-1 receptors must have occurred upon in vitro culture, from at least 2000 receptors (the threshold for detection by FACS) per immature LC to 500 receptors on cultured LC. These data strongly suggest that IL-1 directly affects dendritic cells via functionally high-affinity type I IL-1 receptors and might be critically involved in early events when functionally immature dendritic cells, exemplified by freshly prepared LC, are induced to develop into fully immunostimulatory mature dendritic cells.

CONCLUSION AND OUTLOOK

As outlined in the introduction of this chapter, epidermal LC are members of the dendritic cell system offering the best opportunity to analyze dendritic cells in their different functional states. Based on the above procured data on cytokine-receptor expression by immature dendritic cells exemplified by freshly prepared epidermal LC and after maturation to immunocompetent dendritic cells, the following two conclusions may be drawn.

First, our finding that mature LC/dendritic cells lack M-CSF receptors but express high amounts of GM-CSF binding sites and, in addition, high-affinity type I IL-1 receptors, provides new evidence that dendritic cells constitute a distinct cell lineage of myeloid origin. The dendritic cell lineage clearly deviates from macrophages/monocytes, which express high amounts of M-CSF receptors (>30,000), relatively low numbers of GM-CSF receptors and usually low-affinity type II IL-1 receptors.[62] Since granulocytes, macrophages and dendritic cells all develop from a common progenitor cell,[63] it is of utmost interest how these distinct pathways of myeloid differentiation are regulated. From many studies, GM-CSF has emerged as a crucial cytokine for all steps within the dendritic cell lineage; initially, GM-CSF induces proliferation of dendritic cell progenitor cells,[64] then it guarantees the viability of dendritic cells[11,65] and finally it mediates the maturation of dendritic cell precursors to fully mature dendritic cells.[10,11] Biological responses of cells to GM-CSF are influenced by three factors: the concentration of GM-CSF, the number of GM-CSF receptors expressed on the target cells and the binding affinity of these receptors, which is regulated by the ratio of the α and β subunits of the receptor.[30] We have now identified IL-1 as an important regulator of dendritic cell function by its action on the level of GM-CSF receptor expression on dendritic cells.

This second conclusion is based on our finding that freshly isolated LC, as in vitro equivalents of LC in situ, express many

functional type I IL-1 receptors, which are downregulated upon
in vitro maturation of LC, whereas concomitantly GM-CSF receptors appear in high numbers. Since LC maturation in situ cannot be induced by GM-CSF but can be via injection of IL-1,[66] we
propose the following model of events, depicted in Figure 3.2,
that might lead to onset of LC maturation.

Upon epidermal injury and entry of foreign antigen, IL-1 is
released either as IL-1α from deposits in keratinocytes or as IL-1β
from LC themselves. IL-1 then interacts in a paracrine or autocrine
manner not only with type I IL-1 receptors on keratinocytes,
but also on LC, which now upregulate their GM-CSF receptors
and thereby become responsive to the GM-CSF released from
"activated" keratinocytes.[67] This will finally lead to the GM-CSF-
dependent maturation of LC. In a comparable way, IL-1 might
also be involved in upregulation of GM-CSF receptors on immature dendritic cells in other organs such as lung or mucosa, and

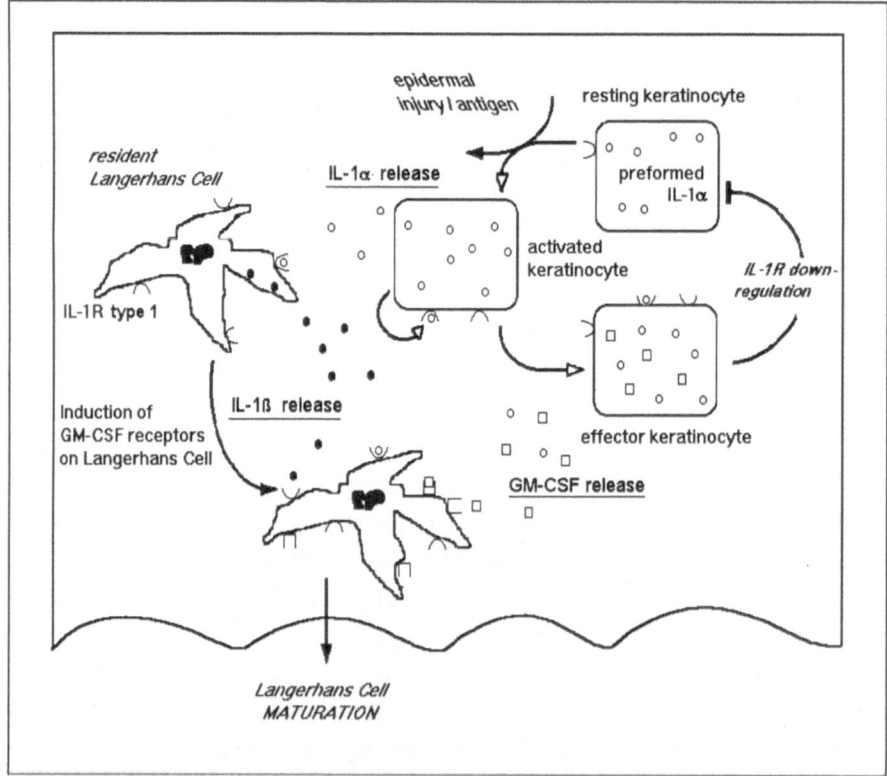

Fig. 3.2. Working model of events within the epidermis that lead to onset of LC maturation.

of course IL-1 will be released during preparation of epidermal cells and induce LC to express GM-CSF receptors in the in vitro situation.

Interestingly, upon intradermal injection, marked differences between IL-1β and IL-1α have been observed in their capacity to induce LC migration and maturation, with IL-1β being far more effective than IL-1α.[68] This discrepancy could recently be confirmed in an organ-culture model system (N. Romani, unpublished data), but is difficult to reconcile at the moment, with the obsevation that IL-1α and IL-1β do act on the same type 1 IL-1 receptor with complete overlapping activities in many cells studied.[52] However, any injected IL-1 will not only directly affect LC, but also induce other cells, e.g., endothelial cells, fibroblasts, melanocytes and especially keratinocytes to react and thereby release several cytokines, including GM-CSF, TNF-α, IL-10, and also antagonists of IL-1 activity such as IL-1Ra or soluble IL-1 receptors. Since IL-1 antagonists such as the membrane and soluble type II IL-1 receptors are far more effective inhibitors of IL-1β than IL-1α, this might result in marked alterations in this complex scenario of cytokines induced by IL-1β and IL-1α and finally account for the observed functional net difference in induction of LC maturation.

This brings us back to the necessity to acquire more knowledge about expression and regulation of LC receptors for cytokines such as TNF-α and IL-10. Furthermore, to better understand the control of epidermal LC maturation, it will be very important to monitor whether triggering of a given receptor on LC might modulate expression of the other cytokine receptors in quantity and binding affinity. Hopefully, such data may also shed light on certain disease situations where alterations of LC functions may be critically involved in the disease process, e.g., in *Leishmania* infections. Studies on LC cytokine receptor expression in susceptible and resistant mouse strains upon infection with *Leishmania major* are currently underway. Ultimately, data on cytokine receptors on dendritic cell precursors at different states of commitment to the dendritic cell lineage and functional maturation might enable us to further optimize the conditions of dendritic cell growth in vitro and probably even to alter the functional capacities of the outgrowing dendritic cells from immunostimulatory towards tolerizing cells.

ACKNOWLEDGMENTS

The support of Prof. Dr. E.-B. Bröcker, Department of Dermatology, Würzburg, is greatly appreciated. This work was supported by the German Science Foundation and by the Austrian Science Foundation (P8549-MED, P9967-MED).

REFERENCES

1. Steinman RM. The dendritic cell system and its role in immunogenicity. Annu Rev Immunol 1991; 9:271-96.
2. Romani N, Witmer-Pack M, Crowley M et al. Langerhans cells as immature dendritic cells. In: Schuler G, ed. Epidermal Langerhans Cells. Boca Raton: CRC Press, 1991:191-216.
3. Romani N, Schuler G. The immunologic properties of epidermal Langerhans cells as a part of the dendritic cell system. Springer Semin Immunopathol 1992; 13:265-79.
4. Schuler G, Steinman RM. Murine epidermal Langerhans cells mature into potent immunostimulatory dendritic cells in vitro. J Exp Med 1985; 161:526-46.
5. Romani N, Koide S, Crowley M et al. Presentation of exogenous protein antigens by dendritic cells to T cell clones: intact protein is presented best by immature epidermal Langerhans cells. J Exp Med 1989; 169:1169-78.
6. Stössel H, Koch F, Kämpgen E et al. Disappearance of certain acidic organelles (endosomes and Langerhans cell granules) accompanies loss of antigen processing capacity upon culture of epidermal Langerhans cells. J Exp Med 1990; 172:1471-82.
7. Kämpgen E, Koch N, Koch F et al. Class II major histocompatibility complex molecules of murine dendritic cells: Synthesis, sialylation of invariant chain, and antigen processing capacity are down-regulated upon culture. Proc Natl Acad Sci USA 1991; 88:3014-8.
8. Inaba K, Steinman RM. Accessory cell-T lymphocyte interactions. Antigen-dependent and -independent clustering. J Exp Med 1986; 163:247-61.
9. Koch F, Kämpgen E, Schuler G et al. Effective enrichment of murine epidermal Langerhans cells by a modified—"mismatched"—panning technique. J Invest Dermatol 1992; 99:803-7.
10. Witmer-Pack MD, Olivier W, Valinsky J et al. Granulocyte/macrophage colony-stimulating factor is essential for the viability and function of cultured murine epidermal Langerhans cells. J Exp Med 1987; 166:1484-98.
11. Heufler C, Koch F, Schuler G. Granulocyte-macrophage colony-stimulating factor and interleukin-1 mediate the maturation of murine epidermal Langerhans cells into potent immunostimulatory dendritic cells. J Exp Med 1988; 167:700-5.
12. Inaba K, Romani N, Steinman RM. An antigen-independent con-

tact mechanism as an early step in T cell-proliferative reponses to dendritic cells. J Exp Med 1989; 170:527-42.

13. Symington FW, Brady W, Linsley PS. Expression and function of B7 on human epidermal Langerhans cells. J Immunol 1993; 150:1286-95.

14. Koch F, Heufler C, Kämpgen E et al. Tumor necrosis factor alpha maintains the viability of murine epidermal Langerhans cells in culture but in contrast to granulocyte/macrophage colony-stimulating factor without inducing their functional maturation. J Exp Med 1990; 171:159-71.

15. Kämpgen E, Koch F, Bröcker E-B et al. Antigen-independent binding of T cells: unique feature of dendritic cells and immunostimulatory epidermal Langerhans cells. In: Wolf K, ed. Proceedings of the Dermatology 2000 meeting. Vienna, London: CCT Healthcare Communications, 1992:190(Abstract).

16. Koch F, Kämpgen E, Trockenbacher B et al. Tumor Necrosis Factor alpha (TNF alpha) induces loss of immunogenic peptides from MHC class II molecules and thus interrupts the antigen presenting function of epidermal Langerhans cells. J Invest Dermatol 1992; 89:510(Abstract).

17. Enk AH, Angeloni VL, Udey MC et al. Inhibition of Langerhans cell antigen-presenting function by IL-10: A role for IL-10 in induction of tolerance. J Immunol 1993; 151:2390-8.

18. Rosenbach T, Czernielewski J, Hecker M et al. Comparison of eicosanoid generation by highly purified human Langerhans cells and keratinocytes. J Invest Dermatol 1990;95:104-7.

19. Cumberbatch M, Fielding I, Kimber I. Modulation of epidermal Langerhans' cell frequency by tumour necrosis factor-alpha. Immunology 1994; 81:395-401.

20. Enk AH, Katz SI. Early molecular events in the induction phase of contact sensitivity. Proc Natl Acad Sci U S A 1992; 89:1398-402.

21. Heufler C, Topar G, Koch F et al. Cytokine gene expression in murine epidermal cell suspensions: Interleukin 1β and macrophage inflammatory protein 1α are selectively expressed in Langerhans cells but are differentially regulated in culture. J Exp Med 1992; 176:1221-6.

22. Vermeer M, Streilein JW. Ultraviolet B light-induced alterations in epidermal Langerhans cells are mediated in part by tumor necrosis factor-alpha. Photodermatol Photoimmunol Photomed 1990; 7:258-65.

23. Grabbe S, Bruvers S, Granstein RD. Effects of immunomodulatory cytokines on the presentation of tumor-associated antigens by epidermal Langerhans cells. J Invest Dermatol 1992; 99:66S-68S.

24. Kimber I, Cumberbatch M. Stimulation of Langerhans cell migration by tumor necrosis factor α (TNF-α). J Invest Dermatol 1992; 99:48S-50S.

25. Enk AH, Saloga J, Becker D et al. Induction of hapten-specific tolerance by interleukin 10 in vivo. J Exp Med 1994; 179: 1397-1402.

26. Kämpgen E, Koch F, Heufler C et al. Understanding the dendritic cell lineage through a study of cytokine receptors. J Exp Med 1994; 179:1767-76.

27. Williams DE, Bicknell DC, Park LS et al. Purified murine granulocyte/macrophage progenitor cells express a high-affinity receptor for recombinant murine granulocyte/macrophage colony-stimulating factor. Proc Natl Acad Sci USA 1988; 85:487-91.

28. Park LS, Martin U, Sorensen R et al. Cloning of the low-affinity murine granulocyte-macrophage colony-stimulating factor receptor and reconstitution of a high-affinity receptor complex. Proc Natl Acad Sci USA 1992; 89:4295-9.

29. Goodall GJ, Bagley CJ, Vadas MA et al. A model for the interaction of the GM-CSF, IL-3 and IL-5 receptors with their ligands. Growth Factors 1993; 8:87-97.

30. Budel LM, Hoogerbrugge H, Pouwels K et al. Granulocyte-macrophage colony-stimulating factor receptors alter their binding characteristics during myeloid maturation through up-regulation of the affinity converting β subunit (KH97). J Biol Chem 1993; 268:10154-9.

31. Park LS, Friend D, Gillis S et al. Characterization of the cell surface receptor for granulocyte-macrophage colony-stimulating factor. J Biol Chem 1986; 261:4177-83.

32. Watanabe Y, Kitamura T, Hayashida K et al. Monoclonal antibody against the common β subunit (β_c) of the human interleukin-3 (IL-3), IL-5, and granulocyte-macrophage colony-stimulating factor receptors shows upregulation of β_c by IL-1 and tumor necrosis factor-α. Blood 1992; 80:2215-20.

33. Wolff R, Healy AT, Crawford RM et al. Detection of messenger RNA for fms in epidermal cell populations enriched for Langerhans cells. Fed Proc 1987; 46:1223(Abstract).

34. Witmer-Pack MD, Hughes DA, Schuler G. et al. Identification of macrophages and dendritic cells in the osteopetrotic (op/op) mouse. J Cell Sci 1993; 104:1021-9.

35. Reid CD, Stackpoole A, Meager A et al. Interactions of tumor necrosis factor with granulocyte-macrophage colony-stimulating factor and other cytokines in the regulation of dendritic cell growth in vitro from early bipotent CD34+ progenitors in human bone marrow. J Immunol 1992; 149:2681-8.

36. Caux C, Dezutter-Dambuyant C, Schmitt D et al. GM-CSF and TNF-α cooperate in the generation of dendritic Langerhans cells. Nature 1992; 360:258-61.

37. Santiago Schwarz F, Divaris N, Kay C et al. Mechanisms of tumor necrosis factor-granulocyte-macrophage colony-stimulating factor-induced dendritic cell development. Blood 1993; 82:3019-28.

38. Kristensen M, Chu CQ, Eedy DJ et al. Localization of tumour necrosis factor-alpha (TNF-alpha) and its receptors in normal and psoriatic skin: epidermal cells express the 55-kD but not the 75-kD TNF receptor. Clin Exp Immunol 1993; 94:354-62.

39. Smith CA, Farrah T, Goodwin RG. The TNF receptor superfamily of cellular and viral proteins: Activation, costimulation, and death. Cell 1994; 76:959-62.

40. Kämpgen E, Gold R, Eggert A et al. Evidence for apoptotic cell death within the dendritic cell system and its modulation by GM-CSF and TNF alpha. Arch Dermatol Res 1994; 286:230(Abstract).

41. Tartaglia LA, Ayres TM, Wong GHW et al. A novel domain within the 55 kd TNF receptor signals cell death. Cell 1993; 74:845-53.

42. Kutsch CL, Norris DA, Arend WP. Tumor necrosis factor-α induces interleukin-1 and interleukin-1 receptor antagonist production by cultured human keratinocytes. J Invest Dermatol 1993; 101:79-85.

43. Macatonia SE, Doherty TM, Knight SC et al. Differential effect of IL-10 on dendritic cell-induced T cell proliferation and IFN-gamma production. J Immunol 1993; 150:3755-65.

44. Péguet-Navarro J, Moulon C, Caux C et al. Interleukin-10 inhibits the primary allogeneic T cell response to human epidermal Langerhans cells. Eur J Immunol 1994; 24:884-91.

45. Taniguchi T, Minami Y. The IL-2/IL-2 receptor system: A current overview. Cell 1993; 73:5-8.

46. Groh V, Tschachler E, Romani N et al. Tac expression by cultured human Langerhans cells. J Invest Dermatol 1986; 87:142(Abstract).

47. Steiner G, Tschachler E, Tani M et al. Interleukin 2 receptors on cultured murine epidermal Langerhans cells. J Immunol 1986; 137:155-9.

48. MacPherson GG, Fossum S, Harrison B. Properties of lymph-borne (veiled) dendritic cells in culture. II. Expression of the IL-2 receptor: Role of GM-CSF. Immunology 1989; 68:108-13.

49. Inaba K, Steinman RM, Witmer-Pack MW et al. Identification of proliferating dendritic cell precursors in mouse blood. J Exp Med 1992; 175:1157-67.

50. Crowley MT, Inaba K, Witmer-Pack M et al. The cell surface of mouse dendritic cells: FACS analyses of dendritic cells from different tissues including thymus. Cell Immunol 1989; 118:108-25(Abstract).

51. Nakamura Y, Russell SM, Mess SA et al. Heterodimerization of the IL-2 receptor β- and γ-chain cytoplasmic domains is required for signaling. Nature 1994; 369:330-3.

52. Dinarello CA. Interleukin-1 and its biologically related cytokines. Adv Immunol 1989; 44:153-206.

53. Mizutani H, Black R, Kupper TS. Human keratinocytes produce but do not process pro-interleukin-1 (IL-1) beta. Different strategies of IL-1 production and processing in monocytes and keratinocytes. J Clin Invest 1991; 87:1066-71.

54. Hannum CH, Wilcox CJ, Arend WP et al. Interleukin-1 receptor antagonist activity of a human interleukin-1 inhibitor. Nature 1990; 343:336-40.

55. Hammerberg C, Arend WP, Fisher GJ et al. Interleukin-1 receptor antagonist in normal and psoriatic epidermis. J Clin Invest 1992; 90:571-83.
56. Slack J, McMahan CJ, Waugh S et al. Independent binding of interleukin-1α and interleukin-1β to type I and type II interleukin-1 receptors. J Biol Chem 1993; 268:2513-24.
57. Sims JE, Gayle MA, Slack JL et al. Interleukin 1 signaling occurs exclusively via the type I receptor. Proc Natl Acad Sci USA 1993; 90:6155-9.
58. Sims JE, Giri JG, Dower SK. The two interleukin-1 receptors play different roles in IL-1 actions. Clin Immunol Immunopathol 1994; 72:9-14.
59. Giri JG, Newton RC, Horuk R. Identification of soluble interleukin-1 binding protein in cell-free supernatants. Evidence for soluble interleukin-1 receptor. J Biol Chem 1990; 265:17416-9.
60. Koide SL, Inaba K, Steinman RM. Interleukin-1 enhances T-dependent immune responses by amplifying the function of dendritic cells. J Exp Med 1987; 165:515-30.
61. Gallis B, Prickett KS, Jackson J et al. Interleukin-1 induces rapid phosphoylation of the interleukin-1 receptor. J Immunol 1989; 143:3235-40.
62. Chizzonite R, Truitt T, Kilian PL et al. Two high-affinity interleukin 1 receptors represent separate gene products. Proc Natl Acad Sci USA 1989; 86:8029-33.
63. Inaba K, Inaba M, Deguchi M et al. Granulocytes, macrophages, and dendritic cells arise from a common major histocompatibility complex class II-negative progenitor in mouse bone marrow. Proc Natl Acad Sci USA 1993; 90:3038-42.
64. Romani N, Gruner S, Brang D et al. Proliferating dendritic cell progenitors in human blood. J Exp Med 1994; 180:83-93.
65. Naito K, Inaba K, Hirayama Y et al. Macrophage factors which enhance the mixed leukocyte reaction initiated by dendritic cells. J Immunol 1989; 142:1834-9.
66. Nylander Lundqvist E, Bäck O. Interleukin-1 decreases the number of Ia+ epidermal dendritic cells but increases their expression of Ia antigen. Acta Derm Venereol 1990; 70:391-4.
67. Kupper TS. The activated keratinocyte: A model for inducible cytokine production by non-bone marrow-derived cells in cutaneous inflammatory and immune responses. J Invest Dermatol 1990; 94:146S-150S.
68. Enk AH, Angeloni VL, Udey MC et al. An essential role for Langerhans cell-derived IL-1β in the initiation of primary immune responses in skin. J Immunol 1993; 150:3698-3704.

CHAPTER 4

THE ROLE OF INTERLEUKIN-1β AND INTERLEUKIN-10 IN LANGERHANS CELL-MEDIATED IMMUNE RESPONSES

Alexander H. Enk, Stephen I. Katz

INTRODUCTION

The importance of cytokines for the induction of immune responses has been demonstrated in various systems for numerous cell types. In skin, keratinocytes serve as rich sources of various cytokines (interleukin (IL) 1, IL-3, IL-6, IL-7, IL-8, IL-10, IL-12, etc.) and growth factors (granulocyte/macrophage colony-stimulating factor (GM-CSF), etc.) known to be important for the induction and inhibition of inflammatory reactions, thereby providing a basis for the highly varied reaction patterns of the "skin immune system."[1] Indeed the complexity of epidermal cytokine production has been demonstrated, especially for the induction of different cytokines by ultraviolet (UV) light and in inflammatory skin diseases such as psoriasis or atopic dermatitis, as well as contact dermatitis.

Until recently, little was known about the effects of various keratinocyte-derived cytokines on epidermal Langerhans cells (LC). The effects of GM-CSF, tumor necrosis factor α (TNF-α), and

The Immune Functions of Epidermal Langerhans Cells, edited by Heidrun Moll.
© 1995 R.G. Landes Company.

IL-1 on LC had been studied by Schuler and Steinman who demonstrated that GM-CSF is important for the growth and maturation of LC into potent inducers of T cell activation in vitro.[2,3] In contrast, TNF-α serves as a survival factor for LC that sustains the viability of the cells in culture, but does not induce the functional maturation of LC, whereas IL-1 is a moderate stimulator of immune functions of LC in vitro, but does not sustain their viability. As all of these studies were performed in vitro, the in vivo effects of cytokines on epidermal LC have remained unknown. For several years our laboratories have been studying the early events governing the induction phase of allergic contact sensitivity, a model that we have been using to define the functions of various constituents of the skin immune system. In this chapter, we review findings that indicate why contact sensitivity is such a useful model for studying primary immune responses in skin in vivo and will describe those factors important for controlling the induction as well as the downmodulation of this system via effects on epidermal LC.

EARLY EVENTS IN CONTACT SENSITIVITY

Numerous studies have demonstrated the importance of skin in the generation of allergic contact dermatitis and other forms of delayed-type hypersensitivity. Macher and Chase[4-6] demonstrated that the induction of allergic contact dermatitis requires the interaction of hapten with peripheral tissues (skin). These studies were very much in keeping with those of Sulzberger[7] who demonstrated that skin was a unique site for sensitization in that when haptens were injected into organs other than skin, specific unresponsiveness ensued. Thus, the immunologic outcome, that is, the degree of sensitization or tolerance, is governed by the influences that the routes and the manner of antigen exposure exert on helper and suppressor subsets of T cells.

LC are critical in the induction of contact sensitivity.[8] Twenty-four hours after hapten application, increased numbers of dendritic cells appear in regional lymph nodes[9] suggesting that LC migrate from skin into the regional lymph nodes and therein present antigen. Indeed, after challenge with electron-dense allergens, LC have been observed in dermal vessels resembling lymphatics, and in draining lymph nodes after intradermal challenge in sensitized animals.[10]

For the past several years, we have studied mechanisms involved in the induction phase of contact sensitivity. Our early studies demonstrated that application of allergen, but not vehicle or irritant control, caused an increased density of major histocompatibility complex (MHC) class II molecules on LC in the epidermis within 24 hours after hapten application, as well as a change in LC morphology.[11] The upregulation of MHC class II was also accompanied by enhanced immunological function of LC. This could be demonstrated in allogeneic, syngeneic, as well as antigen-specific proliferation assays showing that LC derived from allergen-painted skin were more potent accessory cells than LC derived from control-treated skin. The observations of enhanced MHC class II expression and of functional activation of LC in situ by hapten application motivated us to determine whether cytokines might be involved early in the process of LC activation in the epidermis.

As we wanted to study the induction phase of contact sensitivity and we knew that epidermis is a rich source of cytokines and growth factors,[12] we attempted to determine whether proinflammatory cytokines played an important role in the induction process. We determined whether epidermal-derived allergens induced changes in the expression of IL-1α, IL-1β, GM-CSF, TNF-α, interferon-induced protein 10 (IP-10), macrophage inflammatory protein 2 (MIP-2), and interferon-γ (IFN-γ), using β actin as a control. In addition, we utilized MHC class II molecules (I-Aα) as a positive control, as we had already demonstrated that expression of this molecule was enhanced 24 hours after hapten painting of the skin.[11]

We initially performed a time-course study to analyze changes in various epidermal cytokine mRNA levels following application of the allergen trinitrochlorobenzene (TNCB). To detect the signals derived from all epidermal cells (even small populations such as LC), we used a sensitive, quantitative polymerase chain reaction (PCR) method to analyze early signal changes. Within the first hour of allergen application to skin, there was enhanced expression of mRNA signals for IL-1β, TNF-α and IFN-γ. The upregulation of these cytokines was followed by enhanced expression of signals for IP-10 (within two hours of hapten application), MIP-2 and IL-1α (within four hours), as well as I-Aα (within six hours), whereas β-actin signals remained unchanged.[13] When we investigated changes in the first hour after hapten application in more detail, we identified IL-1β as the first cytokine to be upregulated, and this occurred within 15 minutes after hapten application, followed by TNF-α (within 30 minutes) and IFN-γ (within one hour).[13] To determine whether the enhanced expression of the various cytokines assessed was an allergen-specific effect, or whether the application of vehicle control, irritants or tolerogen might result in similar effects, we applied either an allergen (TNCB), a tolerogen (dinitrothiocyanobenzene; DNTB), or an irritant (sodium lauryl sulfate; SLS) to the ears of mice and determined cytokine mRNA expression 4 hours later. Certain cytokines (IFN-γ, GM-CSF and TNF-α) were upregulated rather nonspecifically after application of the vehicle control to the skin. In contrast, signals for IL-1β, IL-1α, MIP-2, IP-10 and I-Aα were induced only following application of allergen. These data were confirmed by using other allergens like dinitrofluorobenzene (DNFB) and dinitrochlorobenzene (DNCB), as well as irritants such as benzalkonium chloride. In aggregate, our studies identified an allergen-specific cytokine pattern in the early induction phase of contact sensitivity.[13]

Cellular depletion experiments using complement-mediated cytolysis demonstrated that epidermal LC were the major sources of IL-1β and I-Aα signals, whereas T lymphocytes contributed the IFN-γ signals. All the remaining cytokine signals, such as IP-10, MIP-2, IL-1α, TNF-α and GM-CSF, were derived from keratinocytes. As enhanced expression of mRNA signals does not necessarily correlate with the release of protein, we assessed cytokine-protein production in the supernatants of hapten-modified and nonmodified epidermal cells. Immunoreactive TNF-α was detected in the eight-hour supernatants from hapten-modified epidermal cells, but not from the supernatants obtained 20 hours after hapten exposure or from untreated epidermal cells. Immunoreactive IFN-γ was not detected at any time. Thymocyte costimulatory activity used to assess IL-1α was enhanced in the supernatants obtained eight hours after hapten treatment. Biological activity could be inhibited by 90% when anti-IL-1α antibodies at 5 μg/ml were added to the thymocyte assay, whereas it was not affected by addition of anti-IL-1β antibodies. These data suggest that most of the IL-1 produced by epidermal cells is IL-1α, whereas the amounts of IL-1β released by LC are probably beyond the detection limits of our bioassay.[13]

Taken together, these data demonstrate that haptens which are capable of inducing allergic contact sensitivity cause selective profound changes in the signal strength of the mRNA of several cytokines. The earliest of these changes is seen in the IL-1β mRNA signal strength that is increased as early as 15 minutes after hapten painting. In cell-depletion assays, it was demonstrated that the IL-1β signal comes almost entirely from epidermal LC and, although our bioassay could not detect IL-1β protein, we assume that the amounts produced by this subpopulation of cells may be undetectable in our assay system. The findings indicate a critical role for LC-derived IL-1β in the induction of primary immune responses in skin. We next attempted to causally link production of IL-1β by LC to epicutaneous sensitization.

THE ROLE OF LANGERHANS CELL-DERIVED INTERLEUKIN-1β IN THE INITIATION OF PRIMARY IMMUNE RESPONSES IN SKIN

As a strategy to identify a causal relationship between production of IL-1β by epidermal LC and the induction of epicutaneous sensitization, we injected 50 ng of recombinant murine IL-1β (rmIL-1β) into the ears of naive mice. Control mice were injected with phosphate-buffered saline (PBS), TNF-α, IL-1α, or sensitized (as described above) with TNCB. Four hours later, epidermal cell suspensions were prepared, the RNA was extracted, and cytokine signals were determined by quantitative PCR as described above. We again analyzed for expression of the cytokines IL-1α, IL-1β, TNF-α, MIP-2, IL-10 and I-Aα, as well as β-actin controls. Whereas PBS injection did not induce significant changes in the epidermal mRNA pattern, injection of TNF-α and IL-1α only induced MIP-2 signals. In contrast, injection of IL-1β or epicutaneous application of TNCB caused almost identical changes in the epidermal mRNA pattern, that is enhanced expression (10- to 200-fold) of MHC class II I-Aα, MIP-2, TNF-α, IL-1α, IL-10 and even IL-1β. The especially dramatic upregulation of LC-derived IL-1β mRNA after IL-1β injection suggests the existence of a potentially important autocrine loop (Fig. 4.1). In addition, the accumulation of MIP-2 mRNA caused by IL-1β or TNCB was much more striking than the accumulation caused by IL-1α or TNF-α. Doses of IL-1α 10 to 50 times higher resulted in changes of the epidermal cytokines qualitatively similar to those caused by IL-1β or TNCB.[14]

In the next series of experiments, we determined whether IL-1β could directly induce changes in keratinocyte-derived cytokines. We stimulated keratinocyte cultures by addition of either PBS, rmIL-1β, rmIL-1α or trinitrobenzenesulfonate (TNBS), extracted the RNA four hours later and performed PCR analysis for the cytokines described above. As a positive control, RNA derived from TNCB-treated epidermis was processed at the same time. MHC class II primers served as PCR control for complete depletion of LC from the keratinocyte cultures. As expected, no MHC class II signal could be detected in the keratinocyte cultures (Fig. 4.2). In addition, although TNBS alone (in the absence of LC) failed to in-

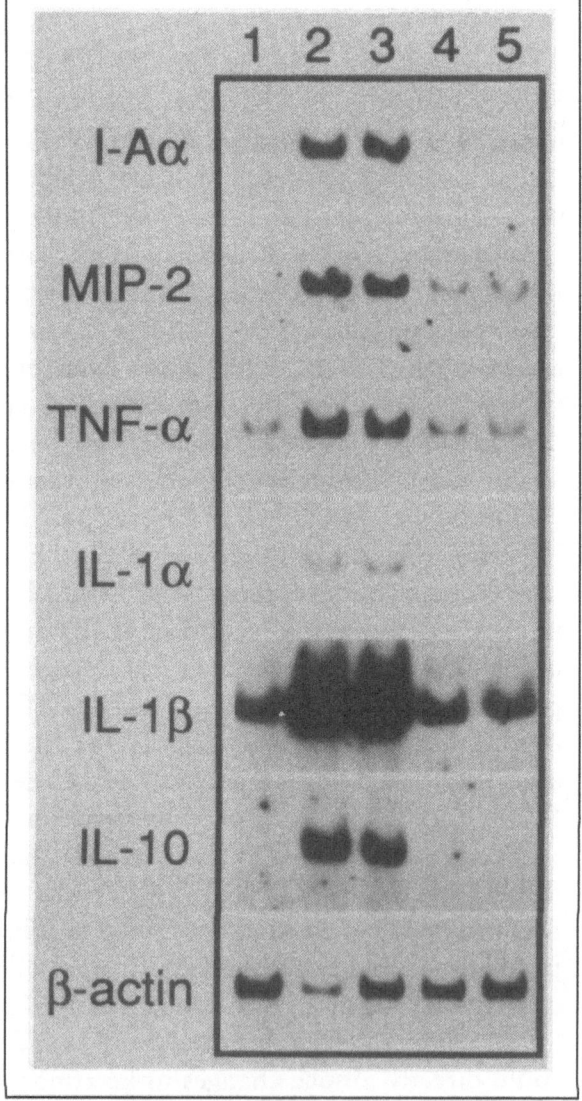

Fig. 4.1. IL-1β injection mimics cytokine mRNA changes induced by contact allergens. Ears of BALB/c mice were injected with 50 μl PBS (lane 1), 50 μl IL-1β (25 ng, lane 2), 50 μl IL-1α (25 ng, lane 4), 50 μl TNF-α (25 ng, lane 5), or 3% TNCB was applied to the skin (lane 3). RNA was extracted 4 hours later as described and analyzed by RT-PCR and liquid hybridization. Reproduced with permission from Enk AH, Angeloni VL, Udey MC et al. J Immunol 1993; 150:3698-704.

duce increased cytokine mRNA signals, IL-1β treatment resulted in a greater than 10-fold increase of MIP-2, TNF-α and IL-10 and a less pronounced (>5-fold) increase of IL-1α mRNA signals (Fig. 4.2). These results mimicked almost exactly the changes induced by in vivo application of TNCB, except for the missing LC-derived MHC class II and IL-1β signals. IL-1α in similar doses had no such effects. These data suggest a crucial role for LC-derived IL-1β in the initiation of subsequent molecular and biologic events in contact sensitivity.[14]

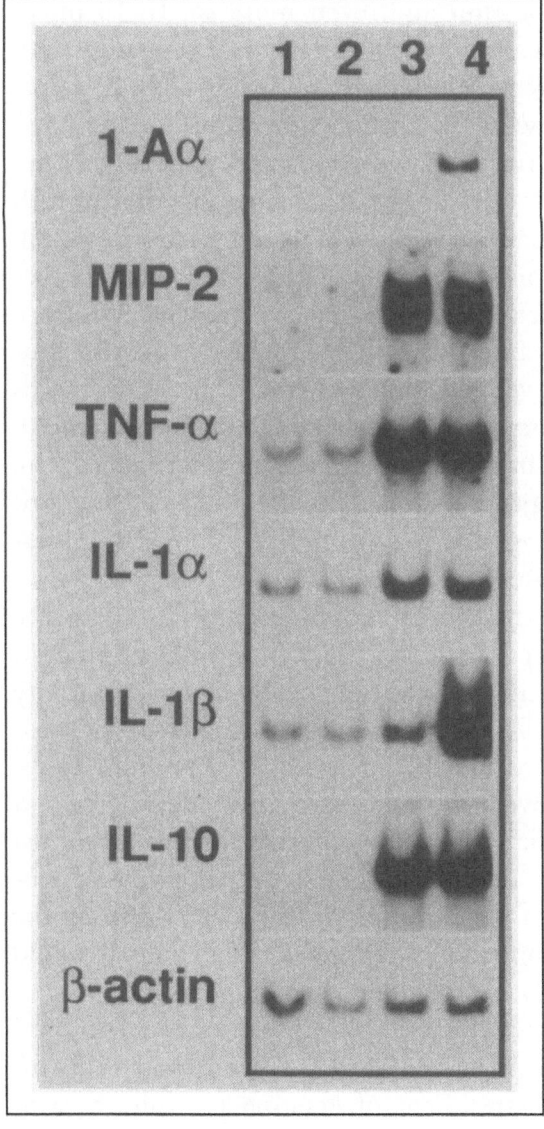

Fig. 4.2. In vitro effects of cytokine or allergen treatment on keratinocyte mRNA signals. LC-free keratinocytes were treated with PBS (lane 1), TNBS (lane 2), and IL-1β (lane 3), or 3% TNCB was applied to the skin (lane 4). Reproduced with permission from Enk AH, Angeloni VL, Udey MC et al. J Immunol 1993; 150: 3698-704.

To determine whether phenotypical changes in the epidermis occurred after injection of IL-1β, we injected 50 ng rmIL-1β, or controls, into the ears of naive mice and prepared epidermal cell suspensions or epidermal sheets 16 hours later. Suspensions as well as sheets were stained with anti-MHC class II monoclonal antibodies (mAb) to identify LC and were analyzed by flow cytometry in a fluorescence-activated cell sorter (FACS) or by fluorescence microscopy (Fig. 4.3). Whereas injection of IL-1α or TNF-α did not cause any changes in the expression of MHC class II molecules or the LC morphology or distribution as compared with PBS-injected skin, TNCB application and, even more so, IL-1β injection caused a dramatic increase in MHC class II expression with the mean fluorescence intensity doubled following TNCB painting, and even tripled following IL-1β injection. Additionally, cells in the IL-1β and TNCB fractions were enlarged in size and decreased in number (<50%). Injection of a blocking anti-IL-1β mAb together with the IL-1β completely prevented the effects of IL-1β.

To address the question of whether LC derived from IL-1β-injected skin were also functionally activated, we prepared LC from epidermis of skin that was injected with IL-1β, IL-1α or PBS four hours after treatment. LC were cocultured with lymph node T cells and anti-CD3 mAb and assessed for their costimulatory potential. Interestingly, LC derived from IL-1β-injected skin were far more potent in inducing T cell proliferation than LC derived from control-treated skin, confirming that LC from IL-1β-injected epidermis are functionally activated.[14]

As a further proof of the critical importance of IL-1β in the induction phase of contact sensitivity, we determined whether it might be possible to prevent sensitization by blocking its activity with a neutralizing mAb. We therefore injected anti-IL-1β or anti-IL-1α neutralizing mAb into the ears of naive mice prior to application of TNCB to the overlying epidermis. Five days later, ear swelling responses were elicited on the contralateral ears. Administration of anti-IL-1β mAb, but not anti-IL-1α mAb, caused virtually complete inhibition of sensitization to TNCB. None of the treatments resulted in the induction of tolerance, as all animals could be subsequently sensitized to TNCB after a short rest period.[14]

Thus, these data emphasize the critical importance of LC-derived IL-1β for the induction of primary immune responses in skin. Injection of IL-1β, as well as treatment of keratinocyte cultures with

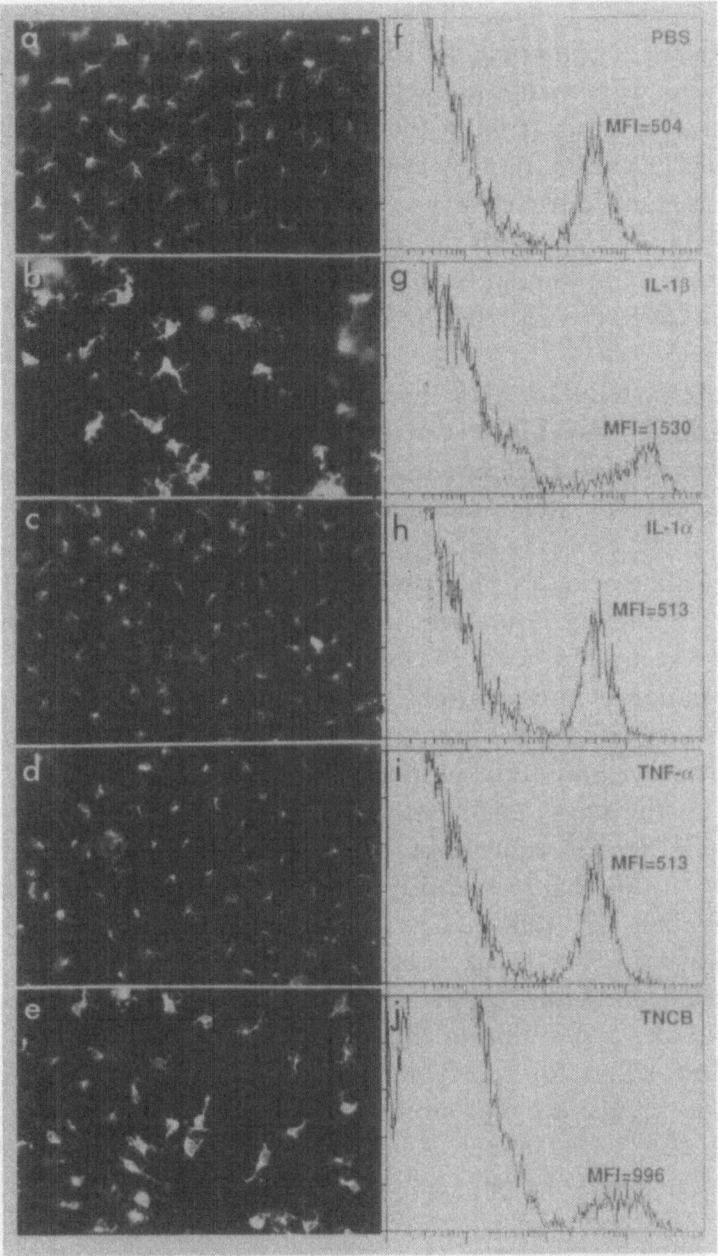

Fig. 4.3. Effect of cytokine injection on epidermal LC. BALB/c mice were injected intradermally with PBS (a and f), 50 ng each of IL-1β (b and g), IL-1α (c and h), TNF-α (d and i), or 3% TNCB was applied (e and j). After 16 hours, either epidermal sheets (left panel) or epidermal cell suspensions (right panel) were prepared and stained for MHC class II expression. MFI = mean fluorescence intensity. Reproduced with permission from Enk AH, Angeloni VL, Udey MC et al. J Immunol 1993; 150:3698-704.

IL-1β, simulates the effects of epicutaneous application of allergen on the epidermal cytokines. In addition, IL-1β caused morphological and phenotypical changes, as well as functional activation of LC similar to, but even more striking than, epicutaneous application of allergen. Finally, anti-IL-1β mAb injection prior to sensitization abrogated the sensitizing capacity of the allergen, proving the essential function of LC-derived IL-1β for the induction of primary immune responses in skin. Similar results on the induction of LC maturation by IL-1 have been reported by Nylander Lundqvist.[15]

INTERLEUKIN-10 AND ITS ROLE IN THE INDUCTION OF TOLERANCE

In most biological systems, inflammatory reactions are usually accompanied by a counterregulatory mechanism. In contact sensitivity, these downregulating effects are depicted by the natural course of the disease with an inflammatory reaction (in mice) peaking at around 24 hours after hapten application and a return to baseline at around 72 to 96 hours. The control of the magnitude and duration of this reaction has been attributed to several factors such as activation of suppressor cells, induction of tolerance, or the release of inhibitory soluble mediators. We were interested in pursuing the latter possibility as, in our initial studies, we had observed that the signals for IFN-γ and IP-10 were upregulated rapidly following the application of allergen, and that this upregulation was followed by the abrupt disappearance of these signals within four to six hours after hapten application although the inflammatory process was ongoing. These findings were, at first, inexplicable. It was during this period that Moore and Mosmann described IL-10 (originally termed cytokine synthesis inhibitory factor) as a molecule that inhibits production of IFN-γ by T helper type 1 (Th1) cell clones.[16,17] Although IL-10 was originally described as a product of Th2 cell clones, we determined whether IL-10 might be released by epidermal cells during the induction phase of contact sensitivity to possibly downmodulate the inflammatory circuit. We detected production of IL-10 mRNA with our sensitive PCR assay.[18] In a time course analysis, we found that IL-10 message was upregulated late in the induction phase as compared with the other proinflammatory cytokines, reaching peak strength only after 12 hours and being downregulated to baseline by 24 hours. This late induction pointed to a possible counterregulatory function of IL-10 in skin. IL-10 mRNA was found to be produced by keratinocytes and its upregulation was found to be specifically induced by contact allergens, as irritants, vehicle or tolerogen failed to induce increased signal strength.[18]

To determine whether IL-10 protein was actually produced by keratinocytes, we again prepared epidermal cell suspensions that were either haptenated or left untreated, and harvested supernatants after metabolic labeling with ^{35}S-methionine for 16 hours. Supernatants were then precipitated with a sensitive solid phase immunoadsorption technique using an IL-10-specific mAb. We detected production of IL-10 protein in the supernatant of haptenated, but not nonhaptenated, epidermal cells.[14] These results were confirmed by Rivas and Ullrich using supernatants from an immortalized keratinocyte cell line (PAM 212) and Western blot analysis.[19]

As IL-10 had been shown to be immunosuppressive via inhibition of antigen-presenting cell (APC) function, we determined the effect of IL-10 on the APC function of LC. Initial experiments demonstrated that IL-10 did not affect anti-CD3 or allogeneic stimulation of naive lymph node T cells supported by LC. We also did not detect any effect of IL-10 on MHC class II expression by LC, in marked contrast to earlier findings in the macrophage system, where IL-10 was shown to inhibit MHC class II expression. However, when assessing T cell proliferation using Th1 or Th2 cell clones, we observed that IL-10 markedly diminished the proliferation of Th1, but not Th2 cell clones, when LC were used as APC. IL-10 effects were more pronounced when LC were preincubated with IL-10 for at least 24 hours. Further studies showed that the effects of IL-10 were independent of antigen processing, as inhibitory effects were seen with both protein- and peptide-pulsed LC.[20]

As it was known from studies with macrophages that IL-10 affected the upregulation of some costimulatory molecules on those cells, we reasoned that cultured LC, known to already express significant numbers of these molecules in comparison to freshly prepared LC, should be resistant to IL-10 effects. Indeed, LC first cultured for three days and then exposed to IL-10 were not inhibited in their accessory functions in Th1 cell proliferation. To further support our hypothesis that IL-10 exerts an inhibitory influence on some costimulator on the surface of LC, we performed an allogeneic costimulator assay using cultured allogeneic LC to supplement for the lack of costimulation on IL-10-treated freshly prepared syngeneic LC.[20] This assay showed that the upregulation of some costimulatory molecule on freshly prepared LC was indeed inhibited by IL-10, and this inhibition was responsible for the deficient APC function of these cells. As lack of costimulation in the presence of antigen presentation, according to Bretscher and Cohn[21] and Schwartz and colleagues,[22] leads to T cell anergy, we determined whether IL-10-treated LC were capable of inducing T cell tolerance in our Th1 cell clone (Fig. 4.4). We found that IL-10-pretreated, but not control-treated LC were capable of inducing anergy in the Th1 clone. Anergy was found to last up to eight days. To exclude a mechanism of cell death, T cells were stimulated with high doses of IL-2, which resulted in good T cell proliferation. In aggregate, our data indicate that IL-10 treatment converts LC from potent immunostimulatory cells to tolerogenic APC in vitro.[20]

To determine whether IL-10 would also be capable of inducing hapten-specific nonresponsiveness in vivo, we next injected 1-2 μg recombinant murine IL-10 (or controls) into the ears of

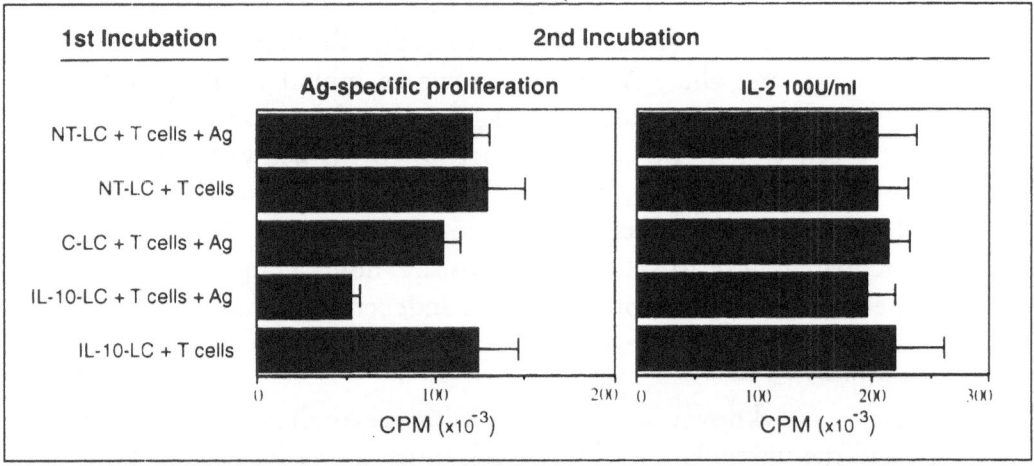

Fig. 4.4. IL-10 treatment renders LC tolerogenic. LC were cultured overnight either in the presence of 100 U/ml IL-10 (IL-10-LC), COS-mock supernatant (C-LC), or with medium alone (NT-LC). Afterwards, epidermal cell suspensions were enriched for LC that were then precultured in 24-well plates with AE7 cells with or without antigen as indicated (first incubation). After 16-20 hours, AE7 cells were rescued and recultured immediately with fresh LC in the presence of antigen (second incubation). The left bars show antigen-specific proliferation, the right bars show T cell responses to 100 U/ml IL-2. Further, T cells precultured in 100 U/ml IL-10 in the absence of LC were fully responsive to subsequent stimulation by LC plus antigen in the absence of IL-10. Background counts for nonrestimulated AE7 cells were 35,000 cpm. Identical results were obtained when the AE7 cells were recultured after resting for one day in complete medium containing 2 U/ml IL-2 (not shown). Reproduced with permission from Enk AH, Angeloni VL, Udey MC et al. J Immunol 1993; 151:2390-7.

mice, eight hours prior to skin application of an allergen (TNCB). Five days later, the contralateral ear was painted with hapten and ear swelling responses were determined. Swelling responses of IL-10-pretreated animals were significantly inhibited as compared with control-treated mice. Simultaneous injection of anti-IL-10 mAb and IL-10 completely abrogated the IL-10 effects. To differentiate between a state of nonresponsiveness and the active induction of tolerance, IL-10-treated animals were again treated with TNCB in the absence of any other treatment. Although IL-10 was not injected during this sensitization protocol, this group of animals showed persisting inhibition of ear swelling as compared to controls. To exclude that the animals in this group were unresponsive to any given stimulus, IL-10-pretreated mice were resensitized with a different allergen, DNFB, in the absence of IL-10. In this case, all mice showed a vigorous ear swelling response excluding immunogical incompetence of these mice. Further studies demonstrated that hapten-specific anergy could also be observed in draining lymph node cells from IL-10-treated mice.[23]

To identify possible mechanisms of action of IL-10 in vivo, we performed quantitative PCR analysis of epidermal RNA derived from IL-10- or control-treated mice following allergen application. We assessed signals for IL-1β, IL-1α, TNF-α and β-actin controls. Injection of IL-10, but not the PBS control, inhibited expression of cytokine mRNA signals for IL-1α, IL-1β, and TNF-α significantly. Coinjection of anti-IL-10 mAb together with IL-10 completely abrogated the effect.[23]

Taken together, these data provide evidence for an important immunoregulatory function of keratinocyte-derived IL-10 in contact sensitivity reactions. IL-10 is expressed comparatively late in the induction phase of contact sensitivity and alters the APC function of LC, most likely by affecting the upregulation of some costimulatory cytokine on these APC. IL-10 converts LC from potent inducers of primary immune reactions to tolerogenic APC in vitro. Additionally, IL-10 exerts tolerizing functions in vivo, possibly by altering the epidermal cytokine milieu.

CONCLUSIONS AND FUTURE PERSPECTIVES

In aggregate, our data demonstrate that contact sensitivity serves as an excellent model for studying not only proinflammatory mechanisms leading via the activation of epidermal LC to the sensitization of naive T cells, but also the counterregulatory, modifying events leading to the termination of inflammatory reactions, thereby preventing tissue damage. We have demonstrated in our experiments that IL-1β subserves the role of an essential mediator of contact sensitivity reaction in that it is produced by the LC itself, even working as an autocrine amplifier of LC activation. We showed that IL-1β is the first cytokine specifically enhanced after allergen stimulation of the cells. Injection of IL-1β mimics the changes caused by application of allergen in that it induces a similar cytokine pattern and causes almost identical phenotypical and morphological changes as epicutaneous allergen application. Functionally, LC derived from IL-1β-injected skin were far more potent accessory cells than LC derived from control-injected skin in an anti-CD3 proliferation assay. Finally, injection of an anti-IL-1β mAb, but not injection of an antibody directed against IL-1α, could block sensitization in mice when injected intradermally before application of allergen. These data demonstrate an essential role for IL-1β in the induction of primary immune responses in skin and for the activation of epidermal LC.

In contrast to these more proinflammatory aspects, our finding that IL-10 is induced late in the induction phase of contact sensitivity provides important clues as to how inflammatory reactions in skin are downregulated. Our studies demonstrate that IL-10 inhibits LC-accessory function for Th1 cells, leaving accessory functions of LC for Th2 cells intact. The effect of IL-10 seems to be mediated by an inhibition of costimulatory molecules expressed on the surface of LC, as could be demonstrated in an allogeneic costimulator assay. In addition, LC exposed to IL-10 were converted from potent inducers of T cell proliferation to tolerizing APC. The tolerance-inducing effect of IL-10 could also be demonstrated in vivo in the murine system. Mice injected with IL-10 intradermally before exposure to hapten were tolerized, an effect that was also demonstrated in regional lymph-node proliferation assays in vitro. As a possible mechanism of action of IL-10, diminished production of IL-1β, IL-1α and TNF-α mRNA could be detected in the epidermis following injection of IL-10 and application of allergen.

Besides being important for the understanding of basic mechanisms of LC activation and the regulation of the cytokine homeostasis in the epidermis, our data provide the basis for potentially important clinical applications. The production of IL-1β by epidermal LC early in the induction phase of contact sensitivity and the finding that there is an allergen-specific cytokine cascade in the epidermis, following the application of hapten, for example, can be exploited and used as an in vitro test system for potential allergens. The use of this assay has been facilitated by the introduction of in vitro culture systems for dendritic cells from peripheral human blood. This provides easy access to dendritic cells at various stages of differentiation and therefore facilitates the use of dendritic cell/LC/ keratinocyte-coculture systems that may be necessary for the induction of an allergen-specific cytokine pattern as seen in vivo.

An even more interesting approach is the use of proliferating dendritic cells for the induction of in vivo tolerance. It may be possible to expose these cells to cocktails of cytokines and convert them to tolerizing APC that could then be used as therapeutic agents for contact sensitivity or even autoimmune diseases. These exciting future perspectives are currently being tested in the laboratory for their possible clinical application.

REFERENCES

1. Luger TA, Schwarz T, eds. Epidermal Cytokines and Growth Factors. New York: Marcel Dekker, 1993.
2. Heufler C, Koch F, Schuler G. GM-CSF and IL-1 mediate the maturation of murine epidermal Langerhans cells into potent immunostimulatory cells. J Exp Med 1988; 167:700-5.
3. Witmer-Pack MD, Olivier W, Valinsky J et al. GM-CSF is essential for the viability and function of cultured murine epidermal Langerhans cells. J Exp Med 1987; 166:1484-95.
4. Landsteiner K, Chase MW. Experiments on the transfer of cutaneous sensitivity to single chemical compounds. Proc Soc Exp Biol Med 1942; 49:688-94.
5. Macher E, Chase MW. Studies on the sensitization of animals with simple chemical compounds. XI. The fate of labeled picryl chloride and DNCB after sensitizating injections. J Exp Med 1969; 129:81-102.
6. Macher E, Chase MW. Studies on the sensitization of animals with simple chemical compounds. XII. The influence of the excision of allergic depots on onset of delayed hypersensitivity and tolerance. J Exp Med 1969; 129:103-18.
7. Sulzberger MB. Arsphenamine hypersensitiveness in guinea pigs. Arch Derm Syph 1930; 22:839-58.
8. Haftek M. Langerhans cells in cutaneous pathology. In: Thivolet J, Schmitt D, eds. The Langerhans Cell. Libbey Eurotext 1988; 172:377-85.

9. Macatonia SE, Knight SC, Edwards AJ et al. Localization of antigen on lymph node dendritic cells after exposure to the contact sensitizer fluorescein isothiocyanate. Functional and morphological studies. J Exp Med 1987; 166:1654-67.

10. Silberberg I, Baer R, Rosenthal AS. The role of Langerhans cells in allergic contact dermatitis. A review of findings in man and guinea pigs. J Invest Dermatol 1976; 66:210-7.

11. Aiba S, Katz SI. Phenotypic and functional characterization of in vivo-activated LC. J Immunol 1990; 145:2791-6.

12. Luger TA. Epidermal cytokines. Acta Derm Venereol 1989; 69:61-7.

13. Enk AH, Katz SI. Early molecular events in the induction phase of contact sensitivity. Proc Natl Acad Sci USA 1992; 89:1398-1402.

14. Enk AH, Angeloni VL, Udey MC et al. An essential role for Langerhans cell-derived IL-1β in the induction of primary immune responses in skin. J Immunol 1993; 150:3698-704.

15. Nylander Lundqvist E, Bäck O. Interleukin-1 decreases the number of Ia⁺ epidermal dendritic cells but increases their expression of Ia antigen. Acta Derm Venereol 1990; 70:391-8.

16. Fiorentino DF, Bond MW, Mosmann TR. Two types of mouse T helper cell. IV. Th2 clones secrete a factor that inhibits cytokine production by Th1 clones. J Exp Med 1989; 170:2081-95.

17. Moore KW, Vieira P, Fiorentino DF et al. Homology of cytokine synthesis inhibitory factor (IL-10) to the Epstein-Barr virus gene BCRFI. Science 1990; 248:1230-4.

18. Enk AH, Katz SI. Identification and induction of keratinocyte-derived IL-10. J Immunol 1992; 149:92-5.

19. Rivas JM, Ullrich SE. Systemic suppression of delayed-type hypersensitivity by supernatants from UV-irradiated keratinocytes. J Immunol 1992; 149:3865-71.

20. Enk AH, Angeloni VL, Udey MC et al. Inhibition of LC-APC function by IL-10. A role for IL-10 in induction of tolerance. J Immunol 1993; 151:2390-7.

21. Bretscher PA, Cohn M. A theory of self-nonself discrimination. Science 1970; 163:1042-9.

22. Schwartz RH. Acquisition of immunologic self-tolerance. Cell 1989; 57:1073-5.

23. Enk AH, Saloga J, Becker D et al. Induction of hapten-specific tolerance by IL-10 in vivo. J Exp Med 1994; 179:1397-1402.

CHAPTER 5

IMMUNOELECTRON MICROSCOPIC ANALYSIS OF MAJOR HISTOCOMPATIBILITY CLASS II EXPRESSION ON HUMAN EPIDERMAL LANGERHANS CELLS

A. Mieke Mommaas, Frits Koning

INTRODUCTION

Paul Langerhans first described the epidermal cell which now bears his name in 1868.[1] It was not until 1973 that the first evidence for the involvement of Langerhans cells (LC) in antigen presentation was published.[2] Since then it has become recognized that they represent a crucial component of the peripheral immune system. Electron microscopic analysis of LC demonstrated that they possess a lobulated, frequently convoluted nucleus, a clear cytoplasm with rough endoplasmic reticulum and a well developed Golgi apparatus, devoid of tonofilaments, desmosomes and melanosomes. Their most distinctive feature at the ultrastructural level, however, is the presence of a cytoplasmic organelle with a rod- or tennis racket-like structure, the Birbeck granule (BG).[3]

The Immune Functions of Epidermal Langerhans Cells, edited by Heidrun Moll.
© 1995 R.G. Landes Company.

Here we will discuss three topics that relate to specific LC function in the skin:

1. The intracellular and cell-surface distribution of major histocompatibility complex (MHC) class II molecules on resting and activated LC in situ and the identification of a MHC class II peptide-loading compartment (called the MIIC) in LC.

2. The putative role of the Birbeck granules in endocytosis, processing and presentation of antigens by LC.

3. The influence of ultraviolet B radiation on LC function.

DISTRIBUTION OF MHC CLASS II MOLECULES ON LANGERHANS CELLS AND IDENTIFICATION OF A PUTATIVE MIIC

In the epidermis, LC are the only cell type that constitutively express MHC class II molecules.[4,5] Intracellularly, these class II molecules bind peptide antigens that result from the degradation of (foreign) exogenous antigens. These MHC class II–peptide complexes are subsequently transported to the cell surface where they can be recognized by CD4+ T cells, leading to specific immune responses. This implies that MHC class II-positive cells (antigen-presenting cells) must possess an intracellular compartment in which newly synthesized class II molecules can associate with degradation products of endocytosed exogenous proteins.[6-8] Also, it may be expected that activation of antigen-presenting cells leads to enhanced MHC class II expression, allowing more efficient presentation of peptide antigens. Recently, an intracellular compartment has been identified in cell lines in which MHC class II molecules, markers of the endosomal/lysosomal system and endocytosed proteins colocalize.[9,10] This compartment, therefore, appears to be the site where MHC class II molecules associate with peptide antigens. Such a compartment, however, has not yet been identified in specialized antigen-presenting cells in situ.

In order to obtain insight into the nature of the compartment in which MHC class II molecules bind peptides in human LC and to study the distribution of class II molecules before and after activation of LC in situ, we applied an immunoelectron microscopic (immuno EM) technique using an MHC class II-specific monoclonal antibody (mAb) conjugated to 10 nm colloidal gold particles on ultrathin cryosections of tissue of normal and acti-

vated human epidermis.[11,12] We found that on normal, unstimulated LC in situ, MHC class II molecules were located on intracellular electron-dense vesicular structures that bear morphological
characteristics of endosomes and lysosomes (Fig. 5.1). Only rarely
could MHC class II be detected on the cell surface of the LC
body. The plasma membrane of the LC dendrites, however, was
always strongly class II-positive (Fig. 5.1). To determine the distribution of MHC class II on activated LC, we used biopsies obtained during the elicitation phase of allergic contact dermatitis
(ACD). We observed that in elicited skin all LC displayed a high
MHC class II expression intracellularly and that class II molecules
were now present on the entire cell surface (Fig. 5.2 and ref. 11).

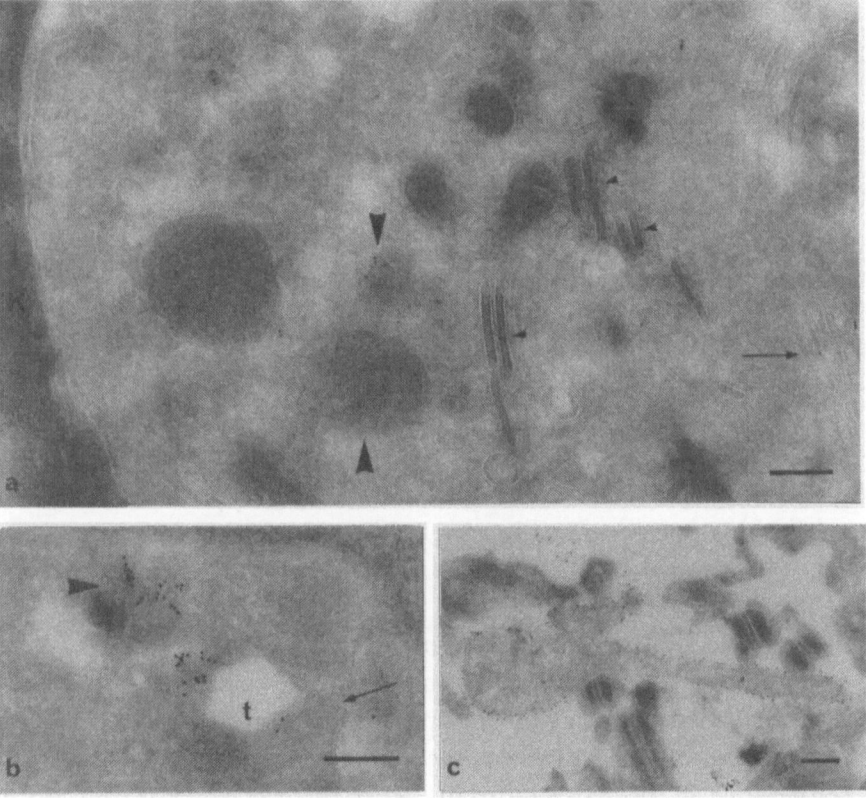

*Fig. 5.1. MHC class II distribution on normal human epidermal LC in situ, visualized by
an MHC class II-specific mAb conjugated to 10 nm colloidal gold applied on ultrathin
cryosections. MHC class II molecules are present in intracellular electron-dense vesicles
(large arrowheads) (a and b), and the Golgi apparatus (small arrows) (a and b), particularly
in the trans-Golgi area (t) (b). The plasma membrane of the cell body is MHC class II-
negative (a), whereas the dendrites show a strong cell-surface MHC class II expression
(c). BG are always class II-negative (small arrowheads). K = keratinocyte. Bar = 0.25 μm.*

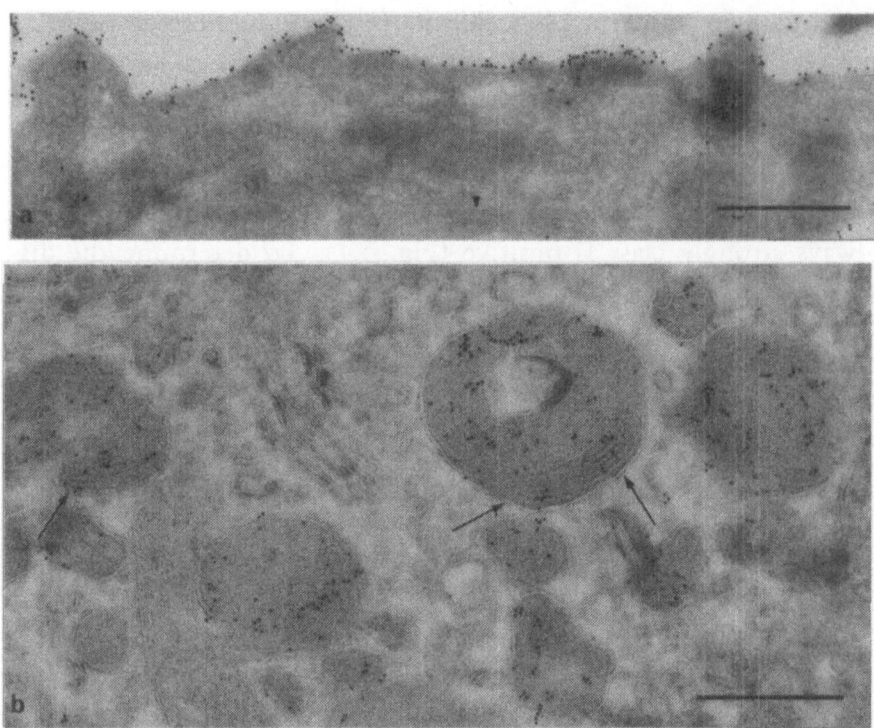

Fig. 5.2. MHC class II expression on human epidermal LC in situ of biopsy specimens of 72-hour positive patch tests, visualized by an MHC class II-specific mAb conjugated to 10 nm colloidal gold applied on ultrathin cryosections. MHC class II molecules have an extensive expression on the cell surface (a) and on intracellular electron-dense vesicles, some of which had a multilaminar structure (arrow) (b). BG are MHC class II-negative (small arrowheads). Bar = 0.5 µm.

Some of the MHC class II-positive vesicles appeared to have a multilaminar structure (Fig. 5.2). These results strongly suggest that activation of LC in situ leads to increased MHC class II synthesis and expression.

Next we analyzed in more detail the nature of the MHC class II-containing intracellular electron-dense vesicles that we found within the LC of both normal and inflamed epidermis (Fig. 5.1A and 5.2B). We performed double-labeling procedures on ultrathin cryosections of human epidermis with the MHC class II-specific mAb conjugated to 10 nm colloidal gold particles, and markers of the endosomal/lysosomal system in conjunction with 5 nm gold. In this way, we established colocalization of MHC class II molecules with Lamp-1, CD63 (not shown), α-glucosidase, and β-hexosaminidase (Fig. 5.3). These vesicles strongly resemble the MIIC

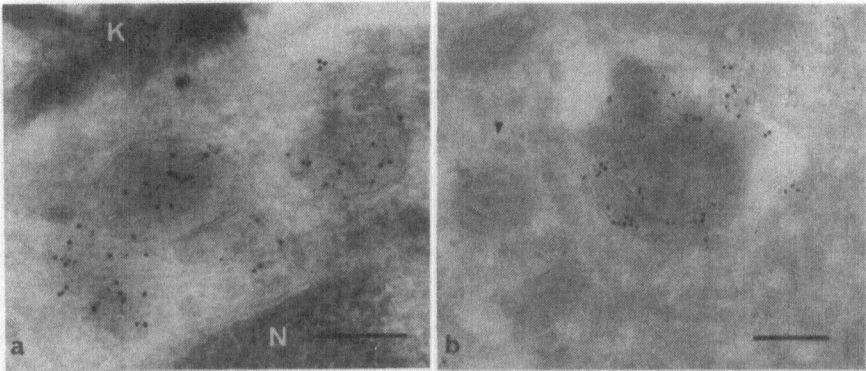

Fig. 5.3. Colocalization in electron-dense vesicles (MIIC) in human epidermal LC in situ of MHC class II molecules, visualized by an MHC class II-specific mAb conjugated to 10 nm colloidal gold and markers of the lysosomal system in conjunction with 5 nm colloidal gold. (a) MHC class II and α-glucosidase, (b) MHC class II and β-hexosaminidase. BG are always negative (small arrowheads). K = keratinocyte, N = nucleus. Bar = 0.25 μm.

first identified by Peters et al in a B cell line[9] and more recently in mouse macrophages and a human melanoma cell line.[13-17]

From these results several conclusions can be drawn:

– Normal, nonactivated human epidermal LC do not constitutively display high cell-surface MHC class II expression on the entire cell surface.

– The surface of the dendrites, however, is strongly MHC class II-positive.

– Activation of LC in situ results in a strong upregulation of MHC class II expression leading to a uniform class II expression on their entire cell surface.

– LC possess a regular MIIC for peptide loading of MHC class II molecules.

The observation that LC do not constitutively express MHC class II products on their entire cell surface is in contrast to the current concept that both murine and human LC express high numbers of MHC class II molecules. This concept is based on previous studies in which MHC class II expression on LC has been determined by immunoperoxidase or immunofluorescence techniques and analysis by light microscopy (LM).[4,5] To determine whether the discrepancy between our results and those previous observations is the result of either the use of different MHC class II-specific antibodies or differences in the staining and analysis techniques employed, we first performed an indirect immunofluorescence/LM analysis of MHC class II expression on LC with the anti-class II antibody we used for our immuno EM experiments. This yielded images similar to those described by others: a diffuse fluorescence on the entire LC suggesting cell-surface labeling of MHC class II molecules (data not shown). Next we applied our immuno EM analysis of MHC class II using freshly *isolated* human epidermal cells. In contrast to the results in situ, strong MHC class II expression was found on the entire cell surface of these isolated LC[18] similar to that found previously by others.[19-22] Together, these results strongly suggest that the discrepancy between our observations and those of others is due to the use of different techniques for visualization of MHC class II molecules. The use of immunoperoxidase or immunofluorescence staining techniques allows diffusion of label, which makes it difficult to exactly determine the location of MHC class II molecules on LC. Moreover, our results indicate that the isolation procedure necessary to obtain a LC suspension results either in the redistribution of MHC class II molecules present on the dendrites (Fig. 5.1), leading to a uniform MHC class II expression on the cell surface, or in activation of LC, resulting in enhanced synthesis and expression of MHC class II. For these reasons, we believe that our observation—that resting LC in situ do not constitutively express MHC class II on their entire cell surface—is an exact reflection of the in vivo situation. In this respect, it is of interest to note that it has recently been shown that immature dendritic cells can be induced to strongly upregulate MHC class II expression in vitro, which results in increased stimulatory capacity in the mixed lymphocyte reaction.[23]

The presence of MHC class II molecules on the dendrites of LC in normal, nonactivated epidermis clearly demonstrates the efficiency of these cells as a reticuloepithelial trap for antigens that gain access to, or arise within the skin. The MHC class II molecules on the dendrites could directly capture and present haptens that do not require internal processing. Subsequently, the induction of a local inflammatory reaction leads to a strong increase in cell surface expression of MHC class II (Fig. 5.2 and refs. 11, 12). Moreover, the enhanced synthesis of MHC class II molecules would favor the association of intracellularly generated peptide antigens with newly synthesized MHC class II molecules, resulting in efficient presentation of exogenous foreign antigens.

Our results indicate that LC possess a specialized compartment in which MHC class II molecules associate with peptide antigens.

Previous studies have demonstrated the presence of such an MIIC compartment in B cells, melanocytes and macrophages.[9,10,13-17] In this acidic compartment, markers for the endosomal/lysosomal system colocalize with MHC class II molecules. It is now well-established that newly synthesized MHC class II molecules associate with the invariant chain in the endoplasmic reticulum and, after passage through the Golgi, are transported to the MIIC.[13] This association with the invariant chain serves at least two purposes: it targets the MHC class II invariant chain complex to the MIIC and it prevents the association of MHC class II molecules with peptides in the endoplasmic reticulum. Removal of the invariant chain is achieved through proteolysis in the MIIC and is thought to expose the peptide-binding site of the MHC class II molecule. Since the MIIC is part of the endosomal/lysosomal system, endocytosed exogenous and membrane antigens are degraded into peptide fragments. These peptide fragments can subsequently bind to MHC class II molecules. Next these MHC class II–peptide complexes are transported to the cell surface. The MIIC is therefore crucial to ensure that MHC class II molecules associate with peptides that are derived from endocytosed (foreign) antigens. The demonstration of the existence of an MIIC in LC indicates that, like other antigen presenting cells, LC use the same pathway for loading of MHC class II with peptides. This is to our knowledge the first demonstration of the existence of such a compartment in a specialized antigen-presenting cell in situ.

ROLE OF BIRBECK GRANULES

Because LC play a crucial role in the elicitation of specific immune responses in the skin, BG have attracted much interest, since they are exclusively found in LC. After the first description of the BG,[3] many papers have addressed the origin and function of this organelle. Some proposed that BG arise in the Golgi area, migrate towards the cell periphery and release their contents into the extracellular space. In the majority of the studies, however, it is suggested that BG originate from the cell membrane and play a role in receptor-mediated endocytosis, intracellular processing and/or presentation of antigens.[20,24-26] It has also been claimed that BG are actively involved in the intracellular traffic of CD1a antigens.[20]

It is well established that BG rapidly disappear from LC upon isolation and culture. Their role in endocytosis, processing and/or presentation is based mostly on electron microscopic studies with LC in situ. Whether or not these organelles play a specific role in LC is therefore still a matter of debate.

When we investigated the localization of CD1a and MHC class II antigens, and markers of the endosomal/lysosomal compartment, we could never find any label on BG (Fig. 5.1 to 5.3 and refs. 11, 12, 18). This suggests that, in contrast to the general opinion, BG do not form part of the endocytic pathway, and do not actively participate in antigen processing and presentation. This possibility was confirmed when we identified a healthy Caucasian 29-year old male, whose LC completely lacked the presence of BG but nevertheless appeared to function normally.[27] Whereas in control individuals approximately 40% of the LC (899 out of 1470, from five individuals) always contained BG, in this particular individual we counted 279 LC, all of which were BG-negative. This was repeatedly observed during a period of three years with five biopsies taken from several areas of the body. The LC of this individual were also not stained by a mAb specific for a BG-associated antigen (Fig. 5.4), confirming the absence of BG in these LC. Despite the complete lack of BG, LC were present in normal numbers, had all the usual morphological characteristics, and were CD1a+ and MHC class II-positive. These BG-negative LC, moreover, displayed normal antigen-presenting capacity: the individual could be sensitized by the hapten diphenylcyclopropenone and this was accompanied by a strong increase in the cell-surface expression of MHC class II antigens on his LC, suggesting LC activation. Furthermore, his epidermal cells elicited a normal positive response in an allogeneic mixed epidermal cell-lymphocyte reaction.[27] These results strongly suggest that BG are not a prerequisite for LC function in vivo and in vitro.

ULTRAVIOLET B-INDUCED IMPAIRMENT
OF LANGERHANS CELL FUNCTION

Ultraviolet B (UVB) radiation has been shown to modify cutaneous immune responses both in animal species and in humans. In mouse skin, UVB treatment impaired the induction of sensitization to dinitrofluorobenzene, and in man it was demonstrated that UVB irradiation could inhibit ACD induction to dinitrochlorobenzene (DNCB).[28,29] The nature of this UVB effect is not fully understood, although it is generally accepted that a reduction in the expression of MHC class II molecules on the LC surface and/or a decrease in the number of LC in the skin is responsible for this effect. To investigate this in more detail we applied our immuno EM technique to study the effect of both short-term and long-term UVB irradiation on MHC class II expression in human epidermis in situ. In addition, the relative number of LC and the morphological features of the epidermis after the UVB protocols were assessed at the ultrastructural level and compared to normal, nonirradiated epidermis.

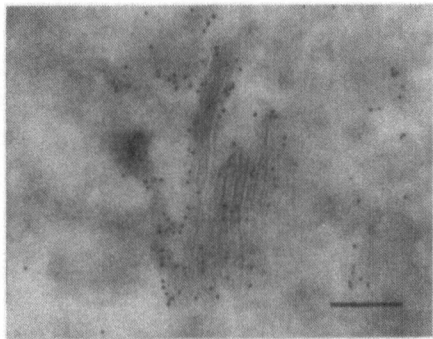

Fig. 5.4. Detail of a normal human epidermal LC stained with a BG-specific mAb and 10 nm colloidal gold, showing labeling of BG. The LC of the BG-negative individual were always negative for this antibody (not shown). Bar = 0.25 μm.

For the short-term studies we employed a low-dose UVB protocol, formerly shown to inhibit the induction of ACD to DNCB.[29] For the long-term effects, a UVB protocol was used that caused a dramatic reduction of the epidermal immune response, assessed by the mixed epidermal cell–lymphocyte reaction.[30] The results of these experiments can be summarized as follows: UVB exposure, either short-term or long-term, did not alter MHC class II expression on human epidermal LC, and although both these UVB protocols were able to cause immune suppression in the skin, these processes were not accompanied by identical morphological features.[12,31,32] After short-term UVB exposure, the epidermal cells (including some LC) exhibited many abnormalities as compared to normal skin. The number of cell layers of the stratum corneum and stratum granulosum was strongly increased. Many cells displayed features of apoptosis such as shrinkage and fragmentation into membrane-bound packages. Furthermore, large vacuoles containing disintegrated cells and neutrophilic granulocytes, and intracellular clefts within the basal cells close to the basal membrane were found. In contrast, after long-term UVB exposure the epidermis had a normal appearance, except for a slight thickening of the stratum corneum. Quantification at the ultrastructural level revealed that after short-term UVB exposure the number of LC had decreased, whereas after long-term UVB exposure the number of LC was similar to normal, untreated epidermis.[12,31,32]

In conclusion, our observations indicate that MHC class II expression is not influenced by UVB treatment. Although with short-term UVB irradiation the number of LC decreased, long-term UVB exposure did not result in decreased number of LC. Moreover, several groups have demonstrated that application of a topical sunscreen or treatment with retinoids prevented LC depletion but did not inhibit short-term UVB-induced immune suppression.[33,34] Thus, local immune suppression is not related to changes in the number of epidermal LC in the skin.

CONCLUSIONS

In summary, we have applied a highly sensitive immunogold-EM technique that allows the exact localization of antigens on the cell surface and on intracellular organelles of cells that are isolated or in situ. With this method, we could demonstrate that normal human epidermal LC in situ do not constitutively display high MHC class II expression on their cell surface, except on the dendrites. This labeling pattern stresses the extreme potential of LC to serve as a reticuloepithelial trap for foreign antigens in the skin. Upon activation, a strong expression of MHC class II appeared on the entire cell surface, suggesting increased synthesis of class II molecules which allows efficient presentation of peptides derived from endocytosed exogenous (foreign) antigens. Loading of such MHC class II molecules with peptides is likely to occur in a specialized compartment, the MIIC. Double labeling of MHC class II and markers of the endosomal/lysosomal compartment indicates that, similar to other antigen-presenting cells, LC possess such an MIIC. BG seem not to be involved in this process. Finally, UVB-induced impairment of LC function appears not to be caused by a reduction of MHC class II expression on LC or by a decreased number of LC in the skin.

Future experiments will focus on the further characterization of the MIIC, in particular the more accurate definition of proteases present in these compartments, which may allow the more precise prediction of peptide epitopes that can be generated in these compartments. Furthermore, we will investigate the putative relationship between the multivesicular and multilaminar MHC class II compartments in LC and the elucidation of their exact role in the generation of functional MHC class II-peptide complexes.

REFERENCES

1. Langerhans P. Über die Nerven der menschlichen Haut. Virch Arch A (Pathol Anat) 1868; 44:325-38.

2. Silberberg I. Apposition of mononuclear cells to Langerhans cells in contact allergic reactions: an ultrastructural study. Acta Derm Venereol 1973; 53:1-12.

3. Birbeck MS, Breathnach AS, Everall JD. An electron microscope study of basal melanocytes and high-level clear cells (Langerhans cells) in vitiligo. J Invest Dermatol 1961; 37:51-64.

4. Rowden G, Lewis MG, Sullivan AK. Ia antigen expression on human epidermal Langerhans cells. Nature 1977; 268:247-8.

5. Klareskog L, Malmnäs Tjernlund U, Forsum U et al. Epidermal Langerhans cells express Ia antigens. Nature 1977; 268:248-50.

6. Harding CV, Unanue ER. Antigen processing and intracellular Ia. Possible roles of endocytosis and protein synthesis in Ia function. J Immunol 1989; 142:12-9.

7. Puré E, Inaba K, Crowley MT et al. Antigen processing by epidermal Langerhans cells correlates with the level of biosynthesis of major histocompatibility complex class II molecules and expression of invariant chain. J Exp Med 1990; 172:1459-69.

8. Davidson HW, Reid PA, Lanzavecchia A et al. Processed antigen binds to newly synthesized MHC class II molecules in antigen-specific B lymphocytes. Cell 1991; 67:105-16.

9. Peters PJ, Neefjes JJ, Oorschot V et al. Segregation of MHC class II molecules from class I molecules in the Golgi complex for transport to lysosomal compartments. Nature 1991; 349:669-76.

10. Harding CV, Geuze HJ. Immunogenic peptides bind to class II MHC molecules in an early lysosomal compartment. J Immunol 1993; 151:3988-98.

11. Mommaas AM, Wijsman MC, Mulder AA et al. HLA class II expression on human epidermal Langerhans cells in situ: upregulation during the elicitation of allergic contact dermatitis. Hum Immunol 1992; 34:99-106.

12. Mommaas AM, Mulder AA, Vermeer M et al. Ultrastructural studies bearing on the mechanism of UVB-impaired induction of contact hypersensitivity to DNCB in man. Clin Exp Immunol 1993; 92:487-93.

13. Neefjes JJ, Ploegh HL. Intracellular transport of MHC class II molecules. Immunol Today 1992; 13:179-84.

14. Amigorena S, Drake JR, Webster P et al. Transient accumulation of new class II MHC molecules in a novel endocytic compartment in B lymphocytes. Nature 1994; 369:113-20.

15. Tulp A, Verwoerd D, Dobberstein B et al. Isolation and characterization of the intracellular MHC class II compartment. Nature 1994; 13:120-6.

16. West MA, Lucocq JM, Watts C. Antigen processing and class II MHC peptide-loading compartments in human B-lymphoblastoid cells. Nature 1994; 13:147-51.

17. Qiu Y, Xu X, Wandinger-Ness A et al. Separation of subcellular compartments containing distinct functional forms of MHC class

II. J Cell Biol 1994; 125:595-605.

18. Vermeer BJ, Mommaas AM, Wijsman MC et al. Ultrastructural localization of HLA-DR and HLA-DQ molecules in Langerhans cells and B cells: an immunoelectronmicroscopic study. Reg Immunol 1988; 1:85-91.

19. Dezutter-Dambuyant C, Schmitt D, Faure M et al. Immunogold technique applied to simultaneous identification of T6 and HLA-DR antigens on Langerhans cells by electron microscopy. J Invest Dermatol 1985; 84:465-8.

20. Hanau D, Fabre M, Schmitt DA et al. Human epidermal Langerhans cells cointernalize by receptor-mediated endocytosis "nonclassical" major histocompatibility complex class I molecules (T6 antigens) and class II molecules (HLA-DR antigens). Proc Natl Acad Sci USA 1987; 84:2901-5.

21. De Panfilis G, Manara GC, Ferrari C et al. Simultaneous colloidal gold immunoelectronmicroscopy labeling of CD1a, HLA-DR, and CD4 surface antigens of human epidermal Langerhans cells. J Invest Dermatol 1988; 91:547-52.

22. Concha M, Vidal A, Garcés G et al. Physical interaction between Langerhans cells and T-lymphocytes during antigen presentation in vitro. J Invest Dermatol 1993; 100:429-34.

23. Sallusto F, Lanzavecchia A. Efficient presentation of soluble antigen by cultured human dendritic cells is maintained by granulocyte/macrophage colony-stimulating factor plus interleukin 4 and downregulated by tumor necrosis factor α. J Exp Med 1994; 179:1109-18.

24. Bartosik J. Cytomembrane-derived Birbeck granules transport horseradish peroxidase to the endosomal compartment in the human Langerhans cells. J Invest Dermatol 1992; 99:53-8.

25. Stössel H, Koch F, Kämpgen E et al. Disappearance of certain acidic organelles (endosomes and Langerhans cell granules) accompanies loss of antigen processing capacity upon culture of epidermal Langerhans cells. J Exp Med 1990; 172:1471-82.

26. Charon CD, Munn CG, Song MJ et al. Internalization of Ia molecules into Birbeck granule-like structures in murine dendritic cells. J Invest Dermatol. 1992; 99:365-73.

27. Mommaas AM, Mulder AA, Vermeer BJ et al. Functional human epidermal Langerhans cells that lack Birbeck granules. J Invest Dermatol 1994; 103:807-10.

28. Toews GB, Bergstresser PR, Streilein JW. Epidermal Langerhans cell density determines whether contact hypersensitivity or unresponsiveness follows painting with DNFB. J Immunol 1980; 124:445-53.

29. Yoshikawa T, Rae V, Bruins-Slot W et al. Susceptibility to effects of UVB radiation on the induction of contact hypersensitivity as a risk factor for skin cancer in humans. J Invest Dermatol 1990; 95:530-6.

30. Van Praag MCG, Out-Luyting C, Claas FHJ et al. Effect of topical sunscreens on the UV-radiation-induced suppression of the alloactivating capacity in human skin in vivo. J Invest Dermatol 1991; 97:629-33.
31. Mommaas AM, Mulder AA, Vermeer BJ. Short-term and long-term UVB-induced immunesuppression in human skin exhibit different ultrastructural features. Eur J Morphol 1993; 31:30-4.
32. Van Praag MCG, Mulder AA, Claas FHJ et al. Long-term ultraviolet B-induced impairment of Langerhans cell function: an immunoelectron microscopic study. Clin Exp Immunol 1994; 95:73-7.
33. Lynch DH, Gurish MF, Daynes RA. Relationship between epidermal Langerhans cell ATPase activity and the induction of contact hypersensitivity. J Immunol 1981; 126:1892-7.
34. Ho KK-L, Halliday GM, Barnetson RSTC. Topical and oral retinoids protect Langerhans cells and epidermal Thy-1⁺ dendritic cells from being depleted by ultraviolet radiation. Immunology 1991; 74:425-31.

CHAPTER 6

ANTIGEN PRESENTATION BY LANGERHANS/DENDRITIC CELLS

Ursula Neiß, Karin Demleitner, Alexandra Marx,
Maria Mehlig, Christoph Scheicher, Konrad Reske

INTRODUCTION

Langerhans cells (LC) intersperse the epidermis forming a thin meshwork of sentinel cells. LC are members of the heterogeneous family of dendritic cells which are recognized to perform an exquisite immunosurveillance function. Distributed throughout the body and localized in nonlymphoid and lymphoid tissues, cells of this category are uniquely equipped to trigger a primary immune response (for review see ref. 1). Notably, processes related to the sentinel function such as antigen uptake and its degradation, and those involving antigen presentation with subsequent T cell priming are separated spacially and by time. Dendritic cells in distinct developmental stages perform these totally different functions. Thus, sentinel dendritic cells such as LC which reside in peripheral nonlymphoid sites are developmentally immature. They carry phenotypic markers of juvenile dendritic cells, i.e., submaximal levels of major histocompatibility complex (MHC) class I, class II and other markers.[1]

Benefiting from their strategic position, LC capture environmental antigens by endocytosis and, in the case of particulate material, by phagocytosis.[2-4] Antigen uptake has dramatic consequences. It initiates intracellular antigen fragmentation, elaborates

The Immune Functions of Epidermal Langerhans Cells, edited by Heidrun Moll.
© 1995 R.G. Landes Company.

long-lived peptide-MHC class II complexes and triggers the LC's egress from the epidermis.[5-7] Dislocation from the epidermal environment favors the developmental and further functional maturation of LC. The LC transform into circulating veiled dendritic cells. In veiled dendritic cells, functions crucial for antigen handling like phagocytosis or processing are shut off or downregulated to basal levels. Similarly, acidic vesicles which are abundant in immature dendritic cells vanish during developmental maturation.[8]

During their migratory phase, dendritic cells prepare themselves by progressive maturation for T cell encounter. Upregulation of adhesion molecules, MHC class II elements and costimulatory markers entails phenotypic changes. These changes enable dendritic cells to approach the T cells in T cell areas within regional lymphoid organs. There they sensitize naive T cells by presenting the peptides they have generated and brought along from the periphery.

Mouse epidermal LC were shown by in vitro culture to undergo phenotypic and functional alterations that mirror their developmental behavior in vivo.[9-13] Since dendritic cell lines were not described until recently,[14] we and others employed the very useful in vitro system to explore the MHC class II synthesis and expression of freshly prepared and short-term cultured mouse[15-17] and rat[18] LC. It should be emphasized that the spatial and temporal segregation of antigen capture in the periphery by immature LC and of peptide presentation in the regional lymphoid tissues by matured dendritic cells requires peptide persistence. Peptides formed by processing of foreign antigen must be preserved and prevented from being exchanged against self peptides when LC mature into highly efficient T cell sensitizing dendritic cells. Our findings suggest that compact-type folding of MHC class II confers longevity to peptide-class II complexes,[18] and that invariant chains might play an auxiliary role in keeping foreign peptides recognizable to memory when dendritic cells cluster quiescent T cells.

FUNCTIONAL PROPERTIES OF FRESHLY ISOLATED AND SHORT-TERM CULTURED LANGERHANS CELLS

We used two assays to reveal the functional capacity of freshly isolated epidermal LC and LC derived from three days of continuous in vitro culture. When irradiated fresh and cultured LC from Lewis rats were cultivated with nylon wool-fractionated allogeneic LEWIS/AVN spleen cells for 72 hours, the capacity of the

LC to stimulate unprimed allogeneic T cells was increased during short-term in vitro culture (Fig. 6.1A). On the other hand, when various numbers of irradiated fresh and cultured LC were incubated with an ovalbumin (OVA)-specific RT1.B^l-restricted T cell clone in the presence of antigen, the freshly isolated LC proved highly effective accessory cells in presenting the nominal antigen OVA (Fig. 6.1B). A three-day preculture diminished the OVA-presenting capacity of the LC. These findings are consistent with similar findings from human and mouse.[1] They strengthen the interpretation that epidermal LC represent immature dendritic cells whose main occupation is to capture and process invading antigen. During short-term in vitro culture, LC differentiate and mature into highly efficient antigen-presenting cells (APC).

EXPRESSION OF THE PROTEOGLYCAN FORM OF THE INVARIANT CHAIN BY LEWIS RAT LANGERHANS CELLS

A certain proportion of the MHC class II-associated invariant γ chain (Ii) exists in a proteoglycan form (Ii-CS), in which a chondroitin-sulfate side chain is linked covalently to the core protein Ii.[19] Ii-CS was described in a recent report to play a significant role in the stimulation of T cell responses.[20] By directly binding to CD44, the hyaluronate receptor,[21] it was suggested to increase APC–T cell adhesion and/or APC–T cell signal exchange. Thus, the possibility existed that LC produce Ii-CS and that part of the enhanced antigen presentation capacity that is seen upon short-term in vitro culture of LC might be attributable to this proteoglycan. To address this possibility, we first examined the synthesis of Ii-CS in Lewis rat spleen cells by labeling spleen cells in the presence of inorganic sulfate ($^{35}SO_4^{2-}$), extracting the cells with nonionic detergent and applying sequential immunoprecipitation. Part of the precipitates were incubated with chondroitinase. Analysis by sodium dodecyl sulfate–polyacrylamide gel electrophoresis (SDS-PAGE) revealed that the proteoglycan form of the invariant chain migrated as a heterogeneous band ranging from 40 to 70 kD (Fig. 6.2A). As the invariant chain proper, Ii-CS was found associated with both isotypic MHC class II complexes RT1.B (OX6)[22] and RT1.D (not shown). Even larger amounts of Ii-CS occurred unlinked to MHC class II. They were precipitable with rat invariant chain-specific monoclonal antibodies (mAb) RG11.[23]

Fig. 6.1. Functional capacity of freshly isolated and short-term cultured LC. (A) Primary allogeneic mixed lymphocyte reaction: various numbers of distinct Lewis rat-derived APC populations were irradiated and cocultured with 5 x 10⁵ nylon wool-fractionated allogeneic LEWIS/AVN spleen cells for 72 hours. The APC were freshly isolated unfractionated epidermal cells (d0 EC; 2.6% MHC class II-positive), panning-enriched LC starting from freshly prepared epidermal cells (d0 LC; 49% MHC class II-positive), LC panning-enriched after one day (d1 LC; 80% MHC class II-positive) or three days of epidermal cell culture in vitro (d3 LC; 87% MHC class II-positive). Spleen cells (SC) were included as control APC. (B) Presentation of protein antigen: various num-

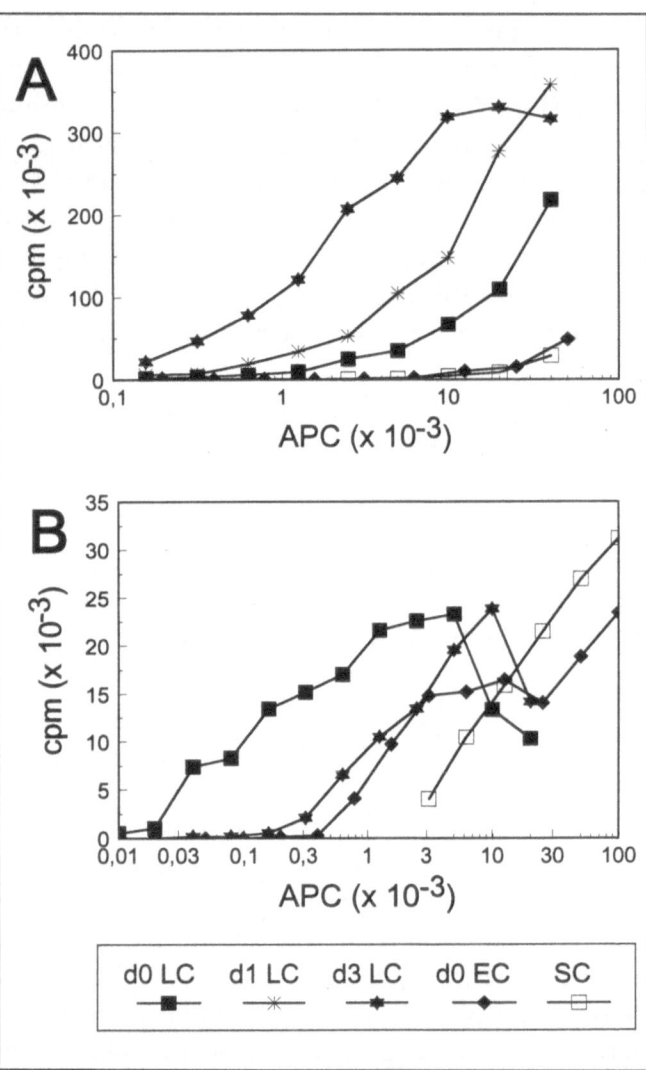

bers of irradiated APC were incubated with 10⁴ cells of the OVA-specific RT1.Bˡ-restricted 1/D6.III T cell clone in the presence of 30 µg/ml OVA. The APC were freshly prepared epidermal cells (d0 EC; 2.3% MHC class II-positive), panning-enriched LC starting from freshly prepared epidermal cells (d0 LC; 37% MHC class II-positive) or following three days of epidermal cell culture (d3 LC; 84% MHC class II-positive) and control spleen cells (SC).

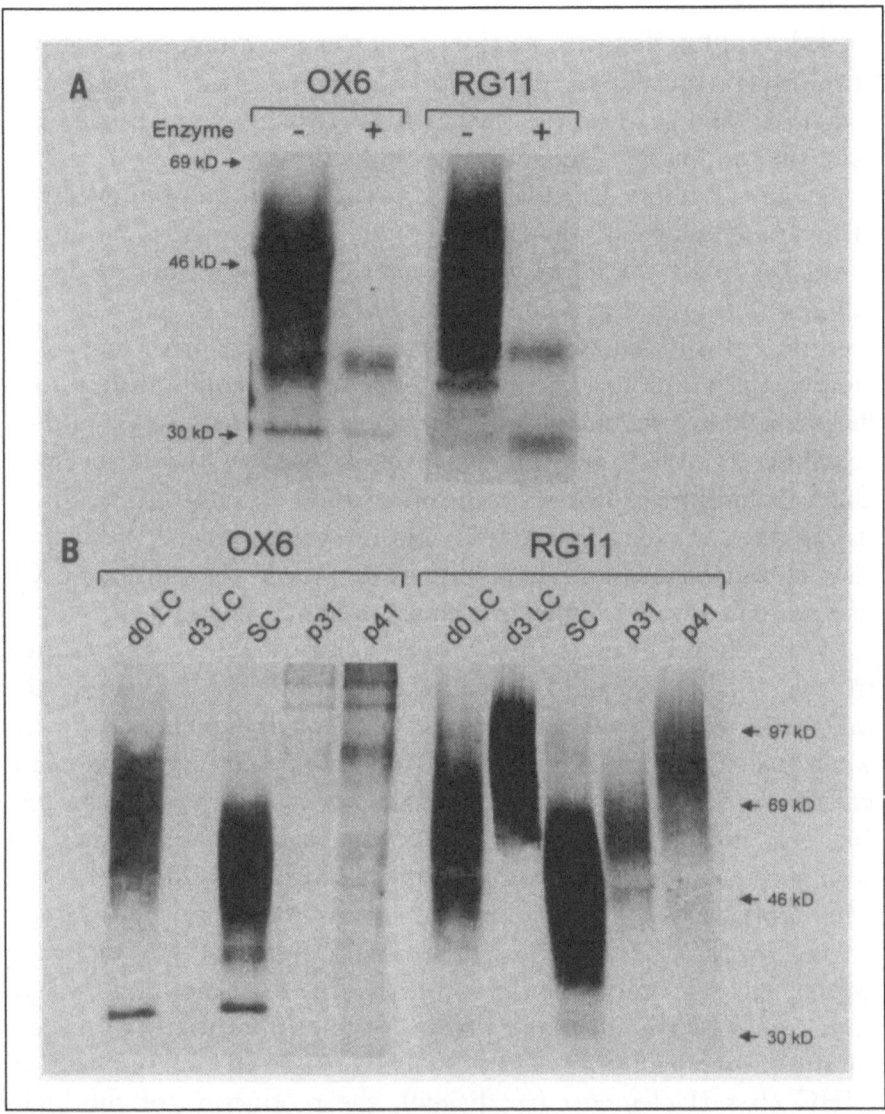

Fig. 6.2. Chondroitin-sulfate form of Ii is synthesized by Lewis rat spleen cells, freshly prepared and three day-cultured LC. (A) Spleen cells were biosynthetically labeled with ^{35}S-sulfate in sulfate-deficient medium. RT1.B-(OX6) and RG11-specific molecules were obtained by sequential immunoprecipitation and resolved by one-dimensional gel electrophoresis (– without, + with, chondroitinase treatment). (B) 2.6 x 10^7 day 0 (d0) LC (49% MHC class II-positive), 1.5 x 10^7 day 3 (d3) LC (87% MHC class II-positive), 2.1 x 10^8 spleen cells, 2.9 x 10^7 p31 COS transfectants and 4.7 x 10^7 p41 COS transfectants were labeled with ^{35}S-sulfate for 4 hours. Proteoglycans were immunoprecipitated by sequentially applying the MHC class II- and invariant chain-specific mAb.

Chondroitinase treatment of MHC class II-associated Ii-CS resulted in almost complete loss of label. The two residual weak bands (MW 30 kD and 35 kD) are likely to belong to trace sulfate-labeled α and β chains. Likewise, the lower molecular weight band of the RG11-specific sample appears to belong to trace-labeled core protein Ii (p31), while the 41-kD band apparently represents the exon 6b-containing alternate splice form of Ii.

Freshly isolated LC (day 0 LC) synthesized substantial levels of invariant chain both in association with MHC class II and in free form (Fig. 6.2B). The broad band of Ii-CS ranges from 46 to 90 kD and thus migrates more slowly than Ii-CS from spleen cells. Cell type-related differences in relative molecular mass have been previously noted and were ascribed to differences in length of the chondroitin sulfate side chain.[20] More importantly, fresh LC exhibited coordinate synthesis and association of MHC class II and invariant chain including its proteoglycan form Ii-CS. By contrast, in three-day cultured LC (day 3 LC), Ii-CS was not coprecipitated with MHC class II, but instead was detectable in free form. In addition, Ii-CS had shifted towards higher molecular weights in day 3 LC.

Since chondroitinase treatment of LC-associated Ii-CS resulted in loss of label, we used a comparative approach to examine the molecular weight shift seen in free Ii-CS of day 3 LC. COS cells were transfected transiently with two Lewis rat invariant chain cDNA clones representing the main invariant chain form p31 (ref. 24) and p41 and were analyzed for proteoglycan synthesis as seen in Figure 6.2B. By comparison, it can be concluded that the core protein of Ii-CS of immature LC is the principal invariant chain form p31. The LC's in vitro maturation has two important consequences for proteoglycan synthesis. The high-molecular weight splice form of the invariant chain, p41, becomes the core protein of the proteoglycan. In addition, in contrast to the synthesis of MHC class II elements (see below), the production of the high-molecular weight form of Ii-CS is maintained in day 3 LC, but p41-CS is not associated with MHC class II. Although further experiments clearly have to be done, in particular studies exploring binding to CD44, these findings are consistent with the notion that the high-molecular weight form of Ii-CS might facilitate dendritic cell–T cell interaction during T cell priming, and that, as suggested earlier,[20] Ii-CS might be responsible for at least part of the stimulatory potential.

UNCOUPLING OF COORDINATE SYNTHESIS OF MHC CLASS II AND INVARIANT CHAINS DURING LANGERHANS CELL CULTURE

We compared the synthesis of MHC class II molecules and invariant chains of freshly prepared and three-day cultured LC by metabolic labeling analysis. In line with their high antigen-processing potential, fresh LC synthesize abundant quantities of MHC class II molecules (Fig. 6.3, day 0 LC). In vitro maturation of LC resulted in a steady decline of MHC class II synthesis to basal levels. Unexpectedly, the synthesis of free invariant chains p31 and p41 increased during in vitro culture to unprecedented levels (Fig. 6.3, RG11). Most importantly, the majority of the free invariant

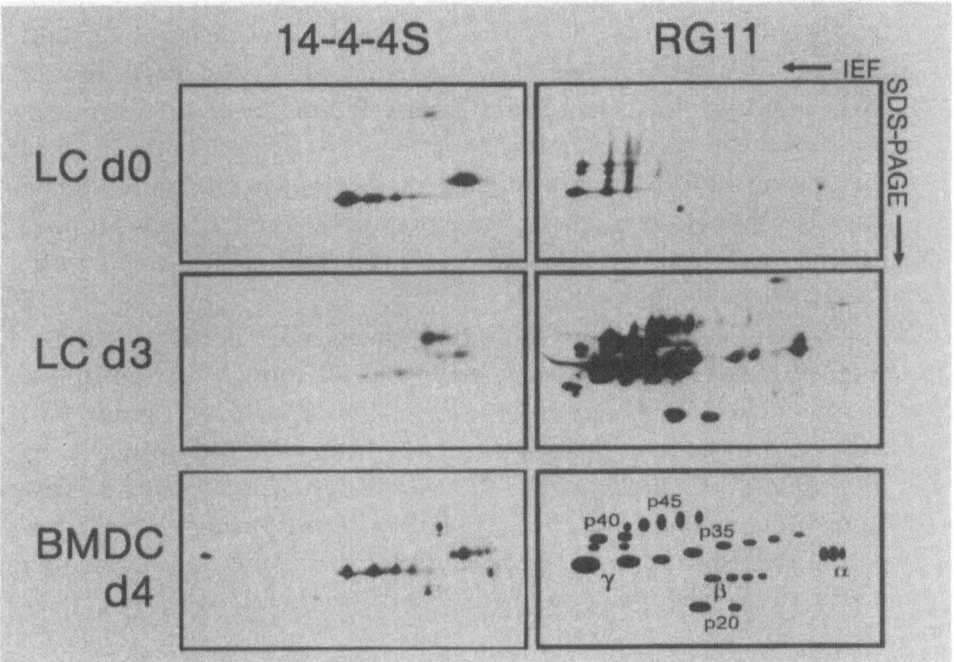

Fig. 6.3. Biosynthetic labeling of panning-enriched LC from freshly isolated and three-day cultured epidermal cell suspensions. 2.4×10^7 enriched fresh LC (d0; 41% MHC class II-positive), 1.7×10^7 three day-cultured LC (d3; 87% MHC class II-positive) and 9.2×10^6 in vitro grown BMDC (day 4; d4) were metabolically labeled for 4 hours in the presence of a mixture of ^{35}S-methionine and ^{35}S-cysteine. Cells were solubilized with NP40 and subjected to sequential immunoprecipitation. Following depletion of the RT1.B-specific molecules, the RT1.D-specific mAb 14-4-4S and the rat invariant chain-specific mAb RG11 were employed. Specific precipitates were resolved by two-dimensional gel electrophoresis. To allow comparison of the amount of newly synthesized proteins by different cell preparations, the gels were exposed to X-ray film for 8 days under identical conditions. Note the prominent levels of mAb RG11-precipitable proteins derived from d3 LC.

chain forms p31 and p41, despite the fact that they are not associated with MHC class II, leave the endoplasmic reticulum and traverse the Golgi compartment. This is evidenced by their prominent sialylation giving rise to terminally glycosylated invariant chain forms designated p35 and p45. Thus the endosomal targeting signal that has been identified in the cytosolic tail of the invariant chains[25,26] appears to be fully operable. In addition, as indicated by the low-molecular weight fragments of the invariant chains, whose quantity increases during the LC's in vitro maturation, the bulk of the terminally glycosylated invariant chains appears to reach the endosomal processing compartment, where it is exposed to catheptic attack.

These findings are remarkable because they clearly document uncoupling of the synthesis of MHC class II and invariant chains in three-day cultured LC, but not in fresh, processing-competent LC. In other MHC class II-synthesizing cell types, regardless of their origin or treatment, MHC class II and invariant chain expression are regulated coordinately. Thus, it appears that in vitro maturation of LC selectively silences the synthesis of new MHC class II elements perhaps because peptide loading, which requires newly synthesized α/β heterodimers in myeloid cells,[27] ought to be prevented in matured LC.

We wished to explore these findings in more detail and, therefore, searched for ways to circumvent the tedious isolation of LC from epidermal cell suspensions. Several groups including our own succeeded in cultivating dendritic cells from bone marrow cells by in vitro culture supplemented with granulocyte/macrophage colony-stimulating factor (GM-CSF).[28,29] Following adaptation of the original procedure to the rat system,[30] we asked the question of whether maturational changes described above for the short-term culture of LC can be seen with bone marrow dendritic cells (BMDC) grown in vitro. Thus, day 4 and day 14 BMDC were subjected to biosynthetic labeling and MHC class II analysis. While day 4 BMDC yielded 14-4-4S (ref. 31) specific precipitates (Fig. 6.3) and RG11-specific precipitates (not shown), whose two-dimensional pattern closely resembled the spot pattern obtained from day 0 LC, a pattern characteristic of day 3 LC with vanishing MHC class II synthesis, but augmented invariant chain synthesis, could not be detected with day 14 BMDC (not shown). We interpret this finding in the light of data from similar studies we are currently performing in the mouse which indicate that a certain proportion of self-renewing progenitors of dendritic cells arises daily during GM-CSF-supplemented bone marrow culture and then develops into MHC class II/Ii-synthesizing immature dendritic cells.

Given the increasing cell-surface expression of MHC class II molecules during in vitro maturation of LC with concomitant decline in MHC class II synthesis, and considering the requirement that peptides occupying the binding groove would have to be preserved during the maturation phase of LC/dendritic cells, we analyzed the MHC class II heterodimers in terms of their resistance to buffer containing sodium dodecyl sulfate (SDS). This convenient assay has been described as distinguishing productive MHC class II-peptide complexes, which exhibit compact-type folding and are therefore SDS-resistant, from other MHC class II associations which fall apart upon treatment with low concentrations of SDS.[32,33] Interestingly, in freshly prepared panning-enriched LC, the majority of the MHC class II elements had acquired the SDS-stable compact-type folding form signaling peptide occupancy.[18] Furthermore, compact-type heterodimers appeared to exhibit peptide-preserving properties because pulse-chase labeling experiments demonstrated that even after three days of continuous LC maturation (chase period 72 hours), precipitable MHC class II molecules consisted almost entirely of compact-type dimers.[18] Again, this is not surprising in the light of the observation that day 3 LC have shut down the synthesis of new MHC class II elements and that in particular newly synthesized MHC class II complexes, comprised of α/β heterodimers in association with invariant chains, are totally SDS-sensitive.

Considering the unprecedented kinetics of the invariant chain synthesis in day 3 LC, we explored the cell surface expression of MHC class II and invariant chains following biotinylation of viable day 3 LC. MHC class II heterodimers of both isotypes (RT1.B; OX6 and RT1.D; 14-4-4S) proved accessible to this type of surface labeling, confirming earlier radio-iodination data. The majority of the two isotypic MHC class II complexes consisted of terminally glycosylated α/β heterodimers (Fig. 6.4). Although small amounts of invariant chains, in particular p41 and its glycosylated form p45, can be detected at the cell surface by RG11 binding, the bulk of the invariant chains, despite being terminally glycosylated (compare Fig. 6.3), appears to be prevented

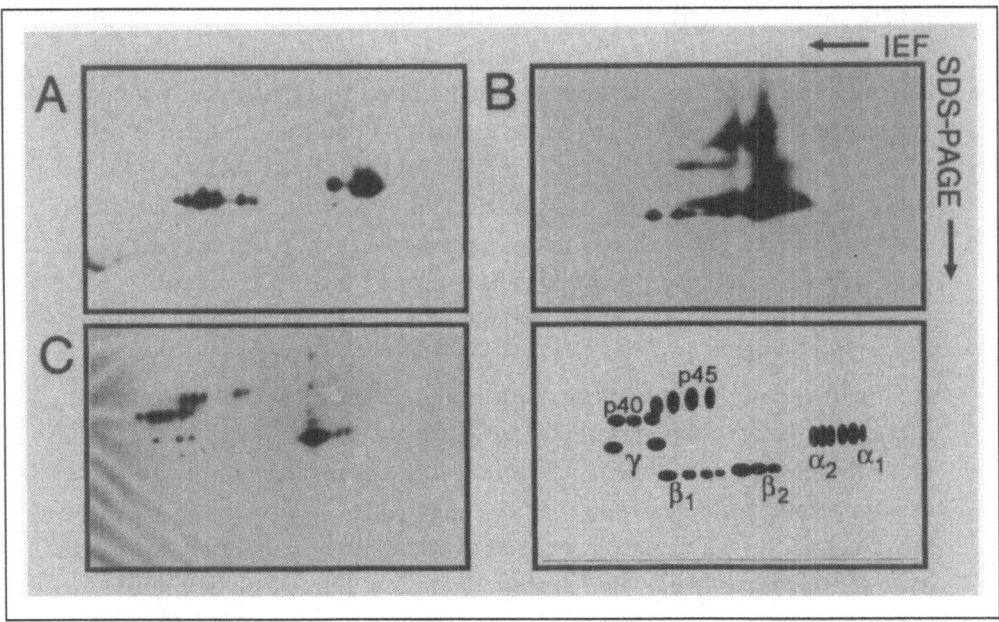

Fig. 6.4. Cell-surface expression of MHC class II molecules on three-day cultured LC. For detection of cell membrane-localized proteins, 3 x 10⁶ enriched LC were cell surface-labeled with activated biotin. Following NP40 extraction, MHC class II molecules were isolated by sequential immunoprecipitation employing mAb OX6 (A), 14-4-4S (B) and RG11 (C). Precipitated proteins were resolved by two-dimensional gel electrophoresis, blotted to a polyvinyldifluoride (PVDF) membrane and were revealed by chemiluminescence detection.

from reaching the cell surface. Its fate seems to be endosomal targeting and degradation.

In summary, sentinel LC, disposed to process invading antigen, mature into migratory veiled dendritic cells and finally into highly efficient peptide-presenting dendritic cells. This development implies at the biosynthesis level a sequence of events that are strictly regulated and that can be envisaged to serve one principal purpose, namely to ensure peptide persistence during the migratory phase of LC/dendritic cells. The continuous synthesis of high levels of invariant chains in the absence of MHC class II production and their poor expression at the cell surface indicate that invariant chains are subject to endosomal degradation and that the high numbers of invariant chain peptides generated might be advantageous for the dendritic cells by curtailing peptide exchange. Several mechanisms for this process can be imagined. The large amounts of invariant chains that enter the endosomal compartment might bind to or modulate endosomal proteases. By competition, this binding could slow down or prevent the generation of peptides from self-proteins that have been taken up by endocytosis. A more straightforward possibility is that invariant chain peptides generated by catheptic proteolysis bind to MHC class II heterodimers which find themselves in a circuit of repetitive cycling. This binding could occur by association with the peptide-binding cleft or by allosteric interaction. In a recent report,[34] it was demonstrated that size-heterogeneous peptides varied greatly in their strength of MHC class II binding, which directly influenced peptide persistence and immunogenicity. Thus, high-affinity binding of appropriately tailored invariant chain peptides, could, either by allosteric interaction or by capping the binding groove, block exchange of foreign against self-peptides. Finally, considering the requirement of the recently described HLA-DM molecules[35,36] for efficient antigen processing, it is also conceivable that the high amounts of invariant chain peptides might interfere with the crucial function of DM.

CONCLUSION

LC and veiled dendritic cells are developmentally interrelated. Both cell types belong to the heterogeneous class of dendritic cells which are destined to perform an immunosurveillance function within the immune system. Three functional phases can be distinguished in the life span of dendritic cells. Juvenile dendritic cells such as epidermal LC residing in nonlymphoid tissues are preoccupied with antigen processing. Following egress from their nonlymphoid environment they head for T cell areas of secondary lymphoid organs and carry with them the peptides they have generated. On their route, they mature and transform to circulating veiled dendritic cells. The hallmark of veiled dendritic cells is peptide transportation. Before the dendritic cells reach their final destination, they undergo profound phenotypic changes. These enable them to trigger an immune response by specifically priming naive T cells.

Withdrawing LC from their dermal environment and placing them into short-term culture induces phenotypic and functional changes that are presumed to reflect the alterations occurring in vivo. We investigated the stimulatory function and MHC class II synthesis including the synthesis of various invariant chain forms in fresh and three day-cultured LC. Fresh LC exhibited vigorous antigen processing as well as MHC class II and invariant chain synthesis, functions that are required for peptide loading. In three-day cultured LC, synthesis of MHC class II elements had ceased, while their cell surface expression was augmented. Most of the MHC class II dimers detected in day 3 LC displayed the compact-type folding state as manifested by SDS resistance. It is suggested that C-type folding of MHC class II dimers confers peptide persistence during developmental maturation of dendritic cells. Notably, synthesis of invariant chains and their posttranslational modification proceeded in three-day cultured LC despite a stop in MHC class II production. This uncoupling of the synthesis of otherwise coordinately regulated elements is postulated to represent a means to ensure peptide persistence. The production of Ii-CS, the chondroitin sulfate-derivatized proteoglycan of the invariant chain, was also shown to be uncoupled from MHC class II synthesis. This finding, together with the identification of the alternately spliced form p41 as the core protein of Ii-CS in day 3 LC, suggests an adhesion molecule-like function of Ii-CS, which in other systems has been described to contribute significantly to T cell stimulation.

ACKNOWLEDGMENTS

This work was supported by the Deutsche Forschungsgemeinschaft, SFB 311, C2 and DARA 50QV9053-6.

REFERENCES

1. Steinman RM. The dendritic cell system and its role in immunogenicity. Annu Rev Immunol 1991; 9:271-96.
2. Inaba K, Inaba M, Naito M et al. Dendritic cell progenitors phagocytose particulates, including Bacillus Calmette-Guérin organisms, and sensitize mice to mycobacterial antigens in vivo. J Exp Med 1993; 178:479-88.
3. Reis e Sousa C, Stahl PD, Austyn JM. Phagocytosis of antigens by Langerhans cells in vitro. J Exp Med 1993; 178:509-19.
4. Scheicher C, Mehlig M, Dienes HP et al. Uptake of bead-absorbed versus soluble antigen by bone marrow-derived dendritic cells triggers their activation and increases their antigen presentation capacity. In: Banchereau J, Schmitt D, eds. Dendritic Cells in Fundamental and Clinical Immunology. New York: Plenum Publishing Corporation, in press.
5. Silberberg-Sinakin I, Thorbecke GJ, Baer RL et al. Antigen-bearing Langerhans cells in skin, dermal lymphatics and in lymph nodes. Cell Immunol 1976; 25:137-51.

6. Larsen CP, Steinman RM, Witmer-Pack M et al. Migration and maturation of Langerhans cells in skin transplants and explants. J Exp Med 1990; 172:1483-93.

7. Kripke ML, Munn CG, Jeevan A et al. Evidence that cutaneous antigen-presenting cells migrate to regional lymph nodes during contact sensitization. J Immunol 1990; 145:2833-8.

8. Stössel H, Koch F, Kämpgen E et al. Disappearance of certain acidic organelles (endosomes and Langerhans cell granules) accompanies loss of antigen processing capacity upon culture of epidermal Langerhans cells. J Exp Med 1990; 172:1471-82.

9. Schuler G, Steinman RM. Murine epidermal Langerhans cells mature into potent immunostimulatory dendritic cells in vitro. J Exp Med 1985; 161:526-46.

10. Shimada S, Caughman SW, Sharrow SO et al. Enhanced antigen-presenting capacity of cultured Langerhans' cells is associated with markedly increased expression of Ia antigen. J Immunol 1987; 139:2551-5.

11. Romani N, Lenz A, Glassel H et al. Cultured human Langerhans cells resemble lymphoid dendritic cells in phenotype and function. J Invest Dermatol 1989; 93:600-9.

12. Streilein JW, Grammer SF. In vitro evidence that Langerhans cells can adopt two functionally distinct forms capable of antigen presentation to T lymphocytes. J Immunol 1989; 143:3925-33.

13. Girolomoni G, Simon JC, Bergstresser PR et al. Freshly isolated spleen dendritic cells and epidermal Langerhans cells undergo similar phenotypic and functional changes during short term culture. J Immunol 1990; 145:2820-6.

14. Paglia P, Girolomoni G, Robbiati F et al. Immortalized dendritic cell line fully competent in antigen presentation initiates primary T cell responses in vivo. J Exp Med 1993; 178:1893-1901.

15. Becker D, Reske-Kunz AB, Knop J et al. Biochemical properties of MHC class II molecules endogenously synthesized and expressed by mouse Langerhans cells. Eur J Immunol 1991; 21:1213-20.

16. Puré E, Inaba K, Crowley MT et al. Antigen processing by epidermal Langerhans cells correlates with the level of biosynthesis of major histocompatibility complex class II molecules and expression of invariant chain. J Exp Med 1990; 172:1459-69.

17. Kämpgen E, Koch N, Koch F et al. Class II major histocompatibility complex molecules of murine dendritic cells: synthesis, sialylation of invariant chain, and antigen processing capacity are down-regulated upon culture. Proc Natl Acad Sci USA 1991; 88:3014-8.

18. Neiß U, Reske K. Non-coordinate synthesis of MHC class II proteins and invariant chains by epidermal Langerhans cells derived from short-term in vitro culture. Intern Immunol 1994; 6:61-71.

19. Sant AJ, Cullen SE, Giacoletto KS et al. Invariant chain is the core protein of the Ia-associated chondroitin sulfate proteoglycan. J Exp Med 1985; 162:1916-34.

20. Naujokas MF, Morin M, Anderson MS et al. The chondroitin sulfate form of invariant chain can enhance stimulation of T cell responses through interaction with CD44. Cell 1993; 74:257-68.

21. Aruffo A, Stamenkovic I, Melnick M et al. CD44 is the principal cell surface receptor for hyaluronate. Cell 1990; 61:1303-13.

22. Fukomoto T, McMaster WR, Williams AF. Mouse monoclonal antibodies against rat major histocompatibility antigens. Two Ia antigens and expression of Ia and class I antigens in rat thymus. Eur J Immunol 1982; 12:237-43.

23. Fisch A, Reske K. Cell surface display of rat invariant γ chain: detection by monoclonal antibodies directed against a C-terminal γ chain segment. Eur J Immunol 1992; 22:1413-9.

24. Henkes W, Syha J, Reske K. Nucleotide sequence of rat invariant gamma chain cDNA clone pLRgamma34.3. Nucleic Acids Res 1988; 16:11822.

25. Bakke O, Dobberstein B. MHC class II associated invariant chain contains a sorting signal for endosomal compartments. Cell 1990; 63:707-16.

26. Lotteau V, Teyton L, Peleraux A et al. Intracellular transport of class II MHC molecules directed by invariant chain. Nature 1990; 348:600-5.

27. Harding CV, Roof RW, Unanue ER. Turnover of Ia-peptide complexes is facilitated in viable antigen-presenting cells: biosynthetic turnover of Ia vs. peptide exchange. Proc Natl Acad Sci USA 1989; 86:4230-4.

28. Scheicher C, Mehlig M, Zecher R et al. Dendritic cells from mouse bone marrow: in vitro differentiation using low doses of recombinant granulocyte-macrophage colony-stimulating factor. J Immunol Meth 1992; 154:253-64.

29. Inaba K, Inaba M, Romani N et al. Generation of large numbers of dendritic cells from mouse bone marrow cultures supplemented with granulocyte/macrophage colony-stimulating factor. J Exp Med 1992; 176:1693-1702.

30. Mehlig M, Scheicher C, Dienes HP et al. Development of rat DC by in vitro culture of bone marrow cells. In: Banchereau J, Schmitt D, eds. Dendritic Cells in Fundamental and Clinical Immunology. New York: Plenum Publishing Corporation, in press.

31. Ozato K, Mayer N, Sachs D. Hybridoma cell lines secreting monoclonal antibodies to mouse H-2 and Ia antigens. J Immunol 1980; 124:533-40.

32. Dornmair K, Rothenhäusler B, McConnel HM. Structural intermediates in the reactions of antigenic peptides with MHC molecules. Cold Spring Harbor Symp Quant Biol 1989; 54:409-16.

33. Germain RN, Hendrix LR. MHC class II structure, occupancy and surface expression determined by post-endoplasmic reticulum antigen binding. Nature 1991; 353:134-9.

34. Nelson CA, Petzold SJ, Unanue ER. Peptides determine the life span of MHC class II molecules in the antigen-presenting cell. Nature 1994; 371:250-2.
35. Fling SP, Arp B, Pious D. HLA-DMA and -DMB genes are both required for MHC class II/peptide complex formation in antigen-presenting cells. Nature 1994; 368:554-8.
36. Morris P, Shaman J, Attaya M et al. An essential role for HLA-DM in antigen presentation by class II major histocompatibility molecules. Nature 1994; 368:551-4.

CHAPTER 7

LANGERHANS CELL MIGRATION: INITIATION AND REGULATION

Ian Kimber, Marie Cumberbatch

INTRODUCTION

Langerhans cells (LC) form a contiguous network within the epidermis. It was proposed by Shelley and Juhlin in 1976[1] that LC represent a trap for external antigens at skin surfaces and since then the role of these cells in cutaneous immune surveillance has excited considerable interest.[2] The theory is that LC act as sentinels of the immune system, sampling the external environment and relaying signals from a potentially hostile antigenic environment to the draining lymph nodes. This phenomenon has been studied extensively within the context of skin sensitization to chemical allergens. In its simplest form the proposal is that following skin sensitization the chemical allergen will associate with resident LC which are then induced to migrate from the skin, via afferent lymphatics, and transport antigen to the draining nodes. To a large extent this sequence of events has been borne out by experimentation.

LANGERHANS CELLS AND SKIN SENSITIZATION

Studies in the mouse have revealed that in response to skin sensitization there is an accumulation of dendritic cells in lymph nodes draining the site of exposure.[3,4] From experiments in which mice were exposed to skin-sensitizing fluorochromes, it is apparent also that a proportion of the dendritic cells which reach drain-

The Immune Functions of Epidermal Langerhans Cells, edited by Heidrun Moll.

ing lymph nodes bear high levels of antigen.[4-6] Evidence that many, if not all, of the dendritic cells which are stimulated to accumulate in skin-draining lymph nodes derive from epidermal LC is provided by several observations. It has been shown that a proportion of the dendritic cells which reach the lymph nodes following skin sensitization contain Birbeck granules, an organelle characteristic of epidermal LC.[7] Moreover, Kripke et al[8] have observed that in nude mice sensitized at the site of an allogeneic skin graft, the antigen-bearing dendritic cells found within draining nodes are of graft donor origin. Nevertheless, it is possible that some dendritic cells, including some antigen-bearing cells, which traffic to nodes following skin sensitization are not of epidermal LC origin.[9] Such cells may derive instead from major histocompatibility complex (MHC) class II (Ia)+ dermal dendritic cells.[10]

LANGERHANS CELL MATURATION

The primary physiological role of dendritic cells is the presentation of antigen. In this respect, the functional activity of LC and their participation in the induction phase of contact sensitivity is intriguing. Freshly isolated epidermal LC are comparatively ineffective antigen-presenting cells. However, the dendritic cells which arrive in lymph nodes, many of which derive from LC, are potent immunostimulatory cells.[2] It is apparent that following skin sensitization and during the process of movement to and entry into the lymph nodes, LC are subject to a functional maturation such that they acquire the antigen-presenting potential characteristic of dendritic cells found within lymphoid tissue. This functional maturation is reflected by phenotypic changes including an important increase in the expression of membrane determinants required for effective interaction with and presentation of antigen to T lymphocytes. Thus, compared with epidermal LC, dendritic cells that arrive in draining lymph nodes display elevated expression of Ia and intercellular adhesion molecule 1 (ICAM-1).[11,12] It is probable also that the migration of LC is associated with increased expression of B7/BB1, a ligand for CD28 and the CD28 homologue CTLA-4, on T lymphocytes and a potent costimulator of CD4+ T cell responses.[13]

There is a general consensus that LC within the skin are able to process antigen effectively and that this facility is lost during migration and the acquisition of antigen-presenting potential.[14]

Consistent with reduced antigen-processing activity is the fact that the maturation of LC is characterized by the loss of Birbeck granules and of endosomal antigens which reflect endocytotic, endosomal and lysosomal activity.[9,15]

It is probable that the changes induced in the phenotype and function of LC are effected by epidermal cytokines. Certainly, cytokines mediate the functional maturation of LC during culture, a process considered analogous to the changes stimulated during the migration of LC in vivo. Of particular importance is granulocyte/macrophage colony-stimulating factor (GM-CSF), a product of keratinocytes.[16] There is no reason to suppose that this cytokine does not exert a similar influence on LC in vivo. Recent evidence indicates that skin cytokines may also provide the stimulus for LC to move away from the epidermis.

LANGERHANS CELL MIGRATION
AND EPIDERMAL CYTOKINES

It is now appreciated that the skin is an immunologically active tissue and that epidermal cells produce constitutively, or can be stimulated to produce, a variety of cytokines. Included among the cytokines synthesized by LC and/or keratinocytes are GM-CSF and other colony-stimulating factors, tumor necrosis factor α (TNF-α), transforming growth factors α and β (TGF-α and TGF-β), macrophage inflammatory proteins 1α and 2 (MIP-1α and MIP-2) and interleukins 1, 6, 7, 8 and 10 (IL-1, IL-6, IL-7, IL-8 and IL-10).[17] We have questioned previously whether one such cytokine, TNF-α, plays a role in LC migration from the epidermis and the accumulation of dendritic cells in draining lymph nodes.

It was found that the intradermal injection of homologous recombinant TNF-α into the ear pinnae of mice caused a rapid accumulation of dendritic cells in draining nodes. Under the same conditions of exposure, intradermal injection of recombinant GM-CSF was without effect. Similarly, injection of bovine serum albumin, the carrier protein administered with TNF-α, failed to influence the number of dendritic cells within draining nodes.[18] The intradermal administration of TNF-α also resulted in a rapid reduction in the frequency of LC local to the site of injection, first apparent within 30 minutes.[19] The tempo of TNF-α-induced changes in the frequency of Ia⁺ epidermal LC and in the numbers of dendritic cells recoverable from draining lymph nodes is illustrated by data from representative experiments displayed in Table 7.1.

An interesting and important observation was that the influence of TNF-α on LC migration and lymph node dendritic cell numbers was species-specific. Intradermal injection of equal amounts of human TNF-α of equivalent specific activity (as judged by cytotoxicity for L929 cells in vitro) failed to induce either a reduction in epidermal LC frequency or the accumulation of dendritic cells in draining lymph nodes (Fig. 7.1).[18,19] It is possible to reconcile such differences on the basis of TNF-α receptor expression. Two distinct receptors for this cytokine are now recognized; a 55-kD form designated TNF-R1 and a 75-kD form, TNF-R2.[20] Human and mouse TNF-R1 exhibit substantial homology in the extracellular domain and, consequently, mouse TNF-R1 has similar affinity for mouse and human TNF-α. In contrast, TNF-R2 is more conserved in the intracellular domain and exhibits weaker homology in the extracellular region resulting in strong species selectivity. Immunocytochemical evidence suggests that epidermal LC express only TNF-R2.[21] It is doubtless for this reason that human TNF-α fails to stimulate LC migration in mice. In contrast to LC, keratinocytes express the 55-kD TNF-R1 form of the

Table 7.1. Influence of intradermal TNF-α on the frequency of Ia⁺ epidermal LC and on the number of dendritic cells within draining lymph nodes

Time following exposure to TNF-α (hours)	Ia⁺ LC/mm² (mean ± SE)	DC/node
0	867.4 ± 26.1	2045
0.5	691.3 ± 37.0	ND
1	739.2 ± 15.2	ND
2	741.3 ± 50.0	3168
4	ND	5313

Groups of BALB/c strain mice received 30 μl intradermal injections into both ear pinnae of 50 ng murine recombinant TNF-α in 0.1% bovine serum albumin. Ears were removed immediately after treatment and at various times thereafter epidermal sheets prepared. The frequency of Ia⁺ LC was measured by indirect immunofluorescence. Results are expressed as the mean number of cells/mm² derived from analysis of 10 fields per sample for each of 4 samples. Lymph node dendritic cells (DC) were enriched and counted following density gradient centrifugation of draining lymph node cell populations on Metrizamide. ND = not done.

receptor.[22] The stimulation of this receptor results in the induction of keratinocyte expression of ICAM-1.[22] Consistent with this is the observation that the intradermal administration to mice of human TNF-α results in the expression by keratinocytes of ICAM-1 under conditions where LC migration is not induced.[19] These data support the heterogeneity of TNF-α receptor expression in the epidermis and also serve to confirm that, in the experiments described above, the failure of human TNF-α to induce LC migration in mice was not attributable to a lack of biologically relevant amounts of the cytokine reaching the epidermis.

A species-selective influence of TNF-α on LC function is suggested also by the results of in vitro experiments. In the course of

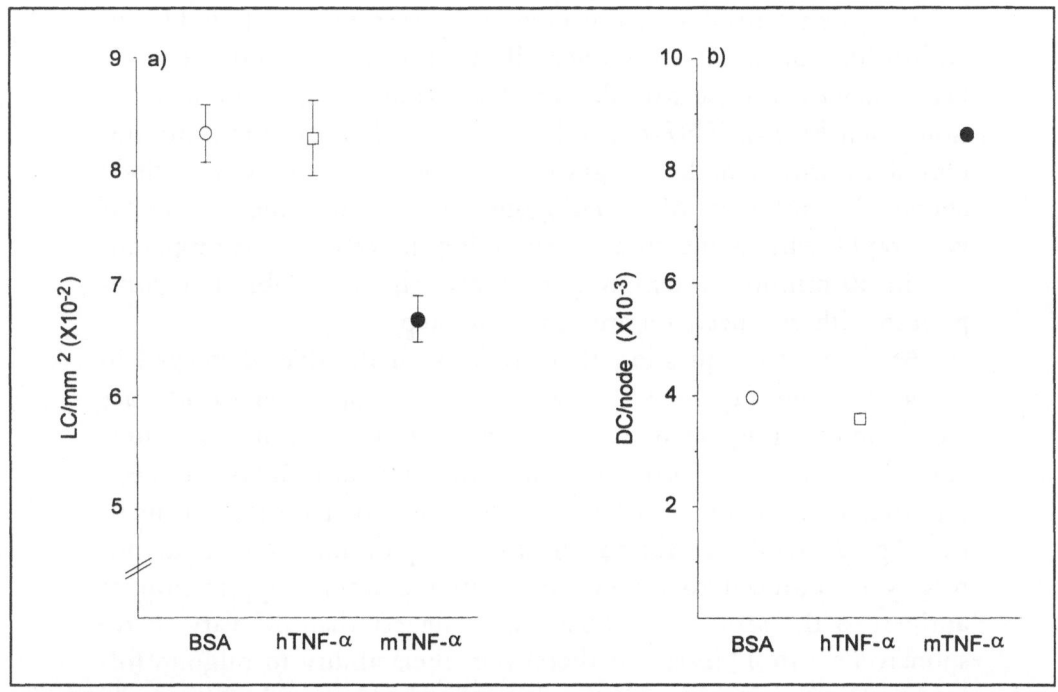

Fig. 7.1. Influence of TNF-α on Langerhans Cell migration and dendritic cell accumulation in draining lymph nodes: a comparison of mouse with human cytokine. Groups of BALB/c strain mice [panel (a) n = 3; panel (b) n = 10] received 30 μl intradermal injections into both ear pinnae of 50 ng human recombinant TNF-α (hTNF-α, □), 50 ng mouse recombinant TNF-α (mTNF-α, ●) or an equal volume of 0.1% bovine serum albumin (BSA, ○) alone. Ears were removed 30 minutes after treatment and epidermal sheets prepared. The frequency of Ia+ LC was measured by indirect immunofluorescence and results expressed as the mean number of cells/mm² derived from analysis of 10 fields per sample for each of four samples (a). Draining lymph nodes were removed 4 hours following treatment. Lymph node dendritic cells (DC) were enriched by density gradient centrifugation on Metrizamide and the number of DC per lymph node estimated by direct morphological examination using phase contrast microscopy (b).

studies designed to investigate the influence of cytokines on LC in culture, it was found that homologous TNF-α served to maintain the viability of the cells without stimulating their functional maturation.[23] Under the same experimental conditions human TNF-α was without effect.[23]

There can be little doubt that the cytokines produced by epidermal cells will individually and in concert orchestrate complex sequences of biological events in the skin and that several act in autocrine and/or paracrine fashion to regulate the synthesis of other cytokines. It is relevant, therefore, to consider whether or not the influence of intradermally administered TNF-α results from a direct effect of the cytokine on resident Langerhans cells. The evidence available indicates that the action of TNF-α is direct. As cited above, a precedent for a direct influence of TNF-α on LC behavior exists insofar as the cytokine serves to maintain LC viability in culture.[23] Moreover, if TNF-α acted indirectly via keratinocytes and the stimulation of keratinocyte cytokine production, then human TNF-α would be expected to exhibit some potential to stimulate LC migration in mice. Finally, as described above, the influence of homologous TNF-α on epidermal LC is very rapid with a measurable reduction in cell density apparent within 30 minutes; a tempo of response which arguably is incompatible with the need for intermediate steps.

An interesting question that arises from the data displayed in Table 7.1 and Figure 7.1 is why only a proportion of LC are stimulated to migrate in response to TNF-α. A similar phenomenon has been described following skin sensitization. It has been reported that for up to 10 days following skin painting, antigen-bearing LC could be found within the epidermis and could not readily be induced to migrate even after a second application of antigen to the same site.[9] These data suggest that LC vary in responsiveness to TNF-α and thereby in their ability to migrate following local exposure to antigen. It may be that such differential behavior is secondary to variable expression of receptors for TNF-α and that LC capable of migrating in response to antigenic challenge or local TNF-α are those that express the highest levels of TNF-R2. Receptor expression may itself be a reflection of maturational status within the skin. There may in fact be a continual low-level migration of LC from the skin to regional lymph nodes providing effective immunological surveillance of the skin even in the absence of overt local trauma or antigen exposure. Possible heterogeneity of TNF-α receptor expression by LC and the relevance of this for migration has yet to be explored.

If TNF-α provides an important signal for LC migration following skin sensitization, then a reduced availability of this cytokine should result in a lower number of dendritic cells reaching the draining lymph nodes. This is borne out by experimentation. It has been demonstrated that systemic administration of anti-TNF-α antibody to mice two hours prior to skin sensitization impaired markedly the accumulation of dendritic cells in draining nodes.[24] Two independent experiments performed using fluorescein isothiocyanate as the sensitizing agent are illustrated in Figure 7.2. The proposal is, therefore, that skin sensitization results in the production, or increased production, by keratinocytes of TNF-α and that this cytokine acts locally on adjacent LC to initiate the process of disengagement from the epidermis and migration to the regional lymph nodes. While it has been shown that topical application of skin-sensitizing chemicals causes the upregulation of TNF-α,[25] there is evidence also that other forms of insult to the skin will similarly stimulate TNF-α production. It is known that topical exposure to sodium lauryl sulphate (SLS), a nonsensitizing skin irritant, and irradiation with ultraviolet B (UVB) light will both enhance TNF-α synthesis.[25,26] Not unexpectedly, therefore, SLS and UVB each induce in mice the accumulation of dendritic cells in draining lymph nodes and in both instances this process can be inhibited significantly by prior treatment with neutralizing anti-TNF-α antibody.[24,27-29] It would appear, therefore, that irrespective of an antigenic challenge, any form of trauma to the skin of sufficient severity and duration to induce TNF-α production will cause the migration of responsive LC from the epidermis. Recognition of this may have important implications for our understanding of UVB light-induced local immunosuppression and of the influence of skin irritation on the efficiency of contact sensitization.[27,29]

In the case of the former, the suggestion is that this ability of UVB irradiation to stimulate the production by keratinocytes of TNF-α will result in a local loss of cytokine-responsive LC. When subsequent challenge with antigen is performed at the same site, there will be insufficient numbers of active LC to respond to this second insult. A role for TNF-α in local immunosuppression by

Fig. 7.2. Influence of anti-TNF-α antibody on the accumulation of dendritic cells in draining lymph nodes following topical exposure to fluorescein isothiocyanate (FITC). Groups of mice (n = 10) received a single 100 μl intraperitoneal injection of either rabbit anti-TNF-α antibody (+) or normal rabbit serum (−). Two hours later, mice were treated on the dorsum of both ears with 25 μl of 1% FITC in 1:1 acetone:dibutylphthalate (ADBP) or with an equal volume of ADBP alone. Draining lymph nodes were removed 18 hours following sensitization and the number of dendritic cells (DC) per lymph node estimated.

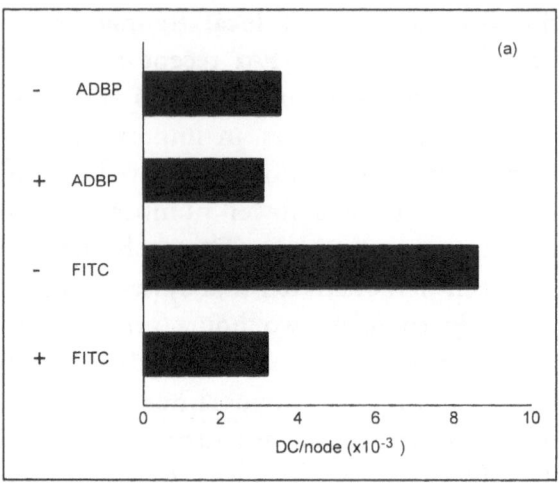

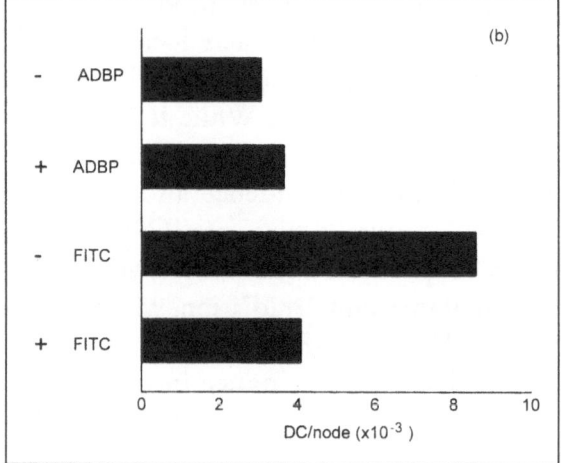

UVB is supported by studies with neutralizing antibody. Systemic administration to mice of anti-TNF-α antibody prior to treatment with UVB was found to reverse the induced local immunosuppression and to restore contact sensitization through the irradiated site to normal levels.[29] The role of local irritation during the induction phase of contact sensitization is of some interest. It has been proposed for many years that skin sensitization is most effective when irritant concentrations of the chemical allergen are applied or when the allergen is applied together with a nonsensitizing skin irritant. The biological basis for the relationship between sensitization and irritation has, however, remained obscure. One possible mechanism is that some degree of skin trauma is necessary to provoke the optimal production by keratinocytes of those cytokines, such as TNF-α and GM-CSF, which effect important changes in LC behavior. The influence of local trauma and epidermal cytokine production is likely to assume greatest significance when chemical allergens are applied at comparatively benign concentrations which do not stimulate a cutaneous inflammatory response.[27]

A case has been developed above for the stimulation of TNF-α production following skin sensitization and for the direct effect of this cytokine on local LC. It is interesting to question whether there exist other intermediary events which are required for, or associated with, TNF-α production after exposure to chemical allergen. It has been proposed that epidermal IL-1β plays an essential role in the induction of contact sensitization. Thus, local injection of anti-IL-1β antibody prevented sensitization to the chemical allergen picryl chloride.[30] There is now available compelling evidence that LC represent the major or exclusive source of IL-1β within the epidermis and that expression of this cytokine is upregulated very rapidly (within 15 minutes) following exposure to skin sensitizing chemicals.[25,30-33] In view of the tempo of IL-1β production following contact sensitization, it is not unreasonable to suppose that increased expression may result directly from interaction of the chemical allergen with epidermal LC, possibly via association with membrane Ia determinants.[34] Whatever the nature of the signals which induce IL-1β production by LC, it is apparent that this cytokine will act locally to effect important changes, including the upregulated expression of other cytokines. Intradermal injection of mice with IL-1β has been found to mimic changes in epidermal cytokine expression associated with skin sensitization, including a substantial increase in mRNA for TNF-α. A unifying hypothesis, therefore, is that contact sensitization stimulates a rapid induction of, or increase in, IL-1β production by LC and that this cytokine acts in paracrine fashion to provoke the synthesis and secretion by keratinocytes of TNF-α. In turn, TNF-α interacts directly with LC to stimulate their migration from the skin. If such a sequence of events is correct, then neutralizing antibodies for IL-1β and TNF-α should each inhibit the induction phase of contact sensitization and this is in fact the case.[24,30] It is suggested also, that IL-1β has important affects upon LC themselves. It has been reported that treatment of the human fibroblastoid cell line SV-80 with IL-1 (or with TNF-α) induces a selective increase in the 75-kD form of the TNF-α receptor.[35] It will be interesting to determine whether the expression by LC of TNF-α receptor is similarly influenced by IL-1β. It has been proposed also that IL-1β may serve to enhance the expression of receptors for (and the response to) GM-CSF by LC.[36] The proposed roles of IL-1β and TNF-α in the stimulation of LC migration are illustrated in Figure 7.3.

THE REGULATION
OF LANGERHANS CELL MIGRATION

If TNF-α provides a signal for LC migration from the skin, then it is relevant to consider the changes this cytokine induces. Certainly, it is likely that the expression by LC and surrounding cells of adhesion molecules will play an important role in this process. It has been demonstrated recently that both LC and keratinocytes display the homophilic adhesion molecule E-cadherin. The suggestion is that reduced expression (by LC and/or keratinocytes) of E-cadherin would allow LC to disassociate themselves from adjacent keratinocytes as an important first step in their migration away from the skin.[37] Consistent with this is evidence that cultured LC express low levels of this molecule and exhibit a reduced affinity for keratinocytes.[37] Also of potential relevance is another

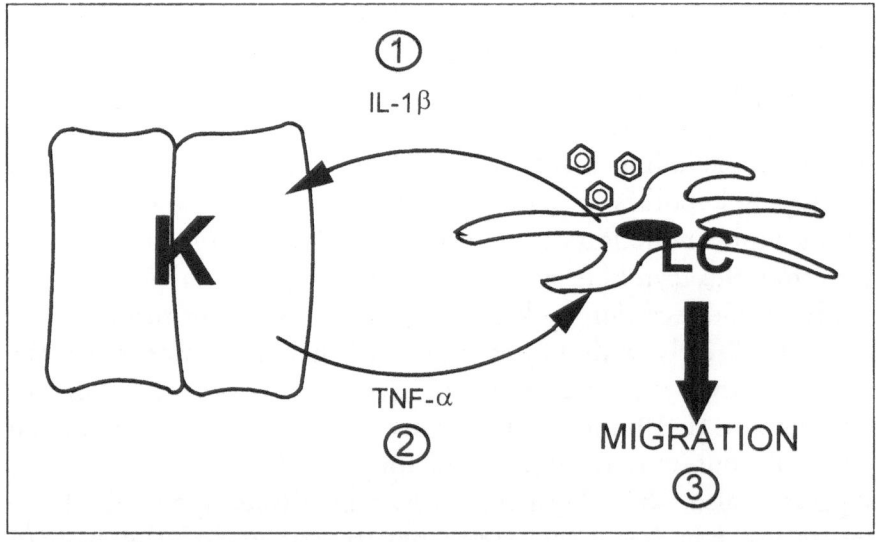

Fig. 7.3. Roles of IL-1β and TNF-α in Langerhans cell migration. Interaction of the chemical allergen with LC induces the upregulation of IL-1β. LC-derived IL-1β acts on adjacent keratinocytes to provoke the production of TNF-α, which in turn stimulates LC migration.

adhesion molecule, CD44, the expression of which has been shown to influence markedly the mobility and migratory activity of various cell types. Significantly, treatment with TNF-α of cultured dendritic cells (which, with respect to surface phenotype, resembled LC) resulted in the increased expression of CD44 and in the appearance of the CD44 exon 9 splice variant (CD44-v9) of this molecule.[38] This latter isoform of CD44 has been associated previously with increased metastatic potential rat carcinoma cells.[39] In a recent investigation it was shown that mice infected with Rauscher leukemia virus display a reduced accumulation of dendritic cells in draining lymph nodes in response to skin sensitization and downregulated expression by epidermal LC of CD44.[40]

Changes in expression of other membrane determinants may also be relevant. Human LC display sialyl Lewis x, a sialylated form of CD15 that serves as a ligand for E-selectin, an adhesion molecule expressed on dermal endothelium. Expression of sialyl Lewis x is enhanced following challenge of nickel-sensitized individuals and it is possible that this molecule facilitates the migration of LC out of the skin.[41,42]

Integrins are collectively a family of widely expressed cell-surface adhesion receptors and represent the major mechanism whereby cells interact with extracellular matrices. Human LC express β1 integrins and it has been proposed that very late antigen (VLA) proteins may allow the adhesion of LC to laminin and fibronectin.[43,44] In mice, LC have been found to possess α4 integrin. Of particular interest is the observation that α4 integrin expression is upregulated markedly during culture of LC and that antigen-bearing cells isolated from the draining lymph nodes of skin-sensitized mice also express this molecule.[45] As a consequence, it has been suggested by Aiba et al[45] that VLA-4 (α4β1 integrins) plays a role in the migration of epidermal LC to the lymph nodes. We are unaware of any evidence that TNF-α serves to influence the expression of α4 integrins by LC. It is the case, however, that TNF-α induces the expression of α6 integrins (α6β4 and α6β1) on human LC.[46] In these studies, it was found that stimulation of mast cell secretion in cultured human neonatal foreskin resulted in α6 expression by LC and the same effect could be achieved by addition of TNF-α, the predominant cytokine within mast cell granules. Moreover, pretreatment of skin cultures with anti-TNF-α antibody prevented the induction of α6 expression in LC by mast cell secretagogues.[46] These data not only demonstrate that TNF-α is able to influence the expression of integrins by LC, but also provides a reminder that cells other than keratinocytes may provide a source of TNF-α during immune and inflammatory responses in the skin.

CONCLUDING COMMENTS

It is proposed that TNF-α provides one signal, and in some instances an exclusive signal, for the migration of LC from the epidermis to draining lymph nodes. It is suggested also that TNF-α interacts directly with TNF-R2 receptors expressed by LC, possibly resulting in the activation of protein kinase C.[47] The nature of the changes induced by TNF-α remains to be elucidated. It is likely, however, that the altered expression by LC (and adjacent cells) of adhesion molecules plays a pivotal role in allowing migration from the skin. Increased availability of TNF-α during skin sensitization and in response to other forms of cutaneous trauma may result from a direct stimulation of keratinocytes (or mast cells) or via the induced secretion by LC of IL-1β.

REFERENCES

1. Shelley WB, Juhlin L. Langerhans cells form a reticuloepithelial trap for external contact allergens. Nature 1976; 261:46-7.
2. Kimber I, Cumberbatch M. Dendritic cells and cutaneous immune responses to chemical allergens. Toxicol Appl Pharmacol 1992; 117:137-46.
3. Knight SC, Krejci J, Malkovsky M et al. The role of dendritic cells in the initiation of immune responses to contact sensitizers. 1. In vivo exposure to antigen. Cell Immunol 1985; 94:427-34.
4. Kinnaird A, Peters SW, Foster JR et al. Dendritic cell accumulation in draining lymph nodes during the induction phase of contact allergy in mice. Int Arch Allergy Appl Immunol 1989; 89:202-10.
5. Macatonia SE, Knight SC. Dendritic cells and the initiation of contact sensitivity to fluorescein isothiocyanate. Immunology 1986; 59:509-14.
6. Cumberbatch M, Kimber I. Phenotypic characteristics of antigen-bearing cells in the draining lymph nodes of contact sensitized mice. Immunology 1990; 71:404-10.
7. Macatonia SE, Knight SC, Edwards AJ et al. Localization of antigen on lymph node dendritic cells after exposure to the contact sensitizer fluorescein isothiocyanate. Functional and morphological studies. J Exp Med 1987; 166:1654-67.

8. Kripke ML, Munn CG, Jeevan A et al. Evidence that cutaneous antigen-presenting cells migrate to regional lymph nodes during contact sensitization. J Immunol 1990; 145:2833-8.

9. van Wilsem EJG, Breve J, Kleijmeer M et al. Antigen-bearing Langerhans cells in skin draining lymph nodes: phenotypes and kinetics of migration. J Invest Dermatol 1994; 103:217-20.

10. Tse Y, Cooper KD. Cutaneous dermal Ia⁺ cells are capable of initiating delayed type hypersensitivity responses. J Invest Dermatol 1990; 94:267-72.

11. Cumberbatch M, Gould SJ, Peters SW et al. MHC class II expression by Langerhans cells and lymph node dendritic cells: possible evidence for maturation of Langerhans cells following contact sensitization. Immunology 1991; 74:414-9.

12. Cumberbatch M, Peters SW, Gould SJ et al. Intercellular adhesion molecule-1 (ICAM-1) expression by lymph node dendritic cells: comparison with epidermal Langerhans cells. Immunol Lett 1992; 32:105-10.

13. Girolomoni G, Zambruno G, Manfredini R et al. Expression of B7 costimulatory molecule in cultured epidermal Langerhans cells is regulated at the mRNA level. J Invest Dermatol 1994; 103:54-9.

14. Streilein JW, Grammer SF. In vitro evidence that Langerhans cells can adopt two functionally distinct forms capable of antigen presentation to T lymphocytes. J Immunol 1989; 143:3925-33.

15. Bucana CD, Munn CG, Song MJ et al. Internalization of Ia molecules into Birbeck granule-like structures in murine dendritic cells. J Invest Dermatol 1992; 99:365-73.

16. Heufler C, Koch F, Schuler G. Granulocyte/macrophage colony-stimulating factor and interleukin 1 mediate the maturation of murine epidermal Langerhans cells into potent immunostimulatory dendritic cells. J Exp Med 1988; 167:700-5.

17. Kimber I. Epidermal cytokines in contact hypersensitivity: immunological roles and practical applications. Toxic In Vitro 1993; 17:295-8.

18. Cumberbatch M, Kimber I. Dermal tumour necrosis factor-α induces dendritic cell migration to draining lymph nodes and possibly provides one stimulus for Langerhans cell migration. Immunology 1992; 75:257-63.

19. Cumberbatch M, Fielding I, Kimber I. Modulation of epidermal Langerhans cell frequency by tumour necrosis factor-α. Immunology 1994; 81:395-401.

20. Lewis M, Tartaglia LA, Lee A et al. Cloning and expression of cDNAs for two distinct murine tumor necrosis factor receptors demonstrate one receptor is species specific. Proc Natl Acad Sci USA 1991; 88:2830-4.

21. Ryffel B, Brockhaus M, Greiner B et al. Tumour necrosis factor receptor distribution in human tissue. Immunology 1991; 74:446-52.

22. Trefzer U, Brockhaus M, Loetscher H et al. 55-kd tumor necrosis factor receptor is expressed by human keratinocytes and plays a pivotal role in regulation of human keratinocyte ICAM-1 expression. J Invest Dermatol 1991; 97:911-6.

23. Koch F, Heufler C, Kämpgen E et al. Tumor necrosis factor α maintains the viability of murine epidermal Langerhans cells in culture, but in contrast to granulocyte/macrophage colony-stimulating factor, without inducing their functional maturation. J Exp Med 1990; 171:159-72.

24. Cumberbatch M, Kimber I. TNF-α is required for accumulation of dendritic cells in draining lymph nodes and for optimal contact sensitization. Immunology 1995; 84:31-5.

25. Enk AH, Katz SI. Early molecular events in the induction phase of contact sensitivity. Proc Natl Acad Sci USA 1992; 89:1398-1402.

26. Kock A, Schwarz T, Kirnbauer R et al. Human keratinocytes are a source for tumor necrosis factor α: evidence for synthesis and release upon stimulation with endotoxin or ultraviolet light. J Exp Med 1990; 172:1609-14.

27. Cumberbatch M, Scott RC, Basketter DA et al. Influence of sodium lauryl sulphate on 2,4-dinitrochlorobenzene-induced lymph node activation. Toxicology 1993; 77:181-91.

28. Moodycliffe AM, Kimber I, Norval M. The effect of ultraviolet B irradiation and urocanic acid isomers on dendritic cell migration. Immunology 1992; 77:394-9.

29. Moodycliffe AM, Kimber I, Norval AM. Role of tumor necrosis factor-α in ultraviolet B light-induced dendritic cell migration and suppression of contact hypersensitivity. Immunology 1994; 81:79-84.

30. Enk AH, Angeloni VL, Udey MC et al. An essential role for Langerhans cell-derived IL-1β in the initiation of primary immune responses in the skin. J Immunol 1993; 150:3698-704.

31. Matsue H, Cruz Jr PD, Bergstresser PR et al. Langerhans cells are the major source of mRNA for IL-1β and MIP-1α among unstimulated mouse epidermal cells. J Invest Dermatol 1992; 99:537-41.

32. Schreiber S, Kilgus O, Payer E et al. Cytokine pattern of Langerhans cells isolated from murine epidermal cell cultures. J Immunol 1992; 149:3525-34.

33. Heufler C, Topar G, Koch F et al. Cytokine gene expression in murine epidermal cell suspensions: interleukin 1β and macrophage inflammatory protein 1α are selectively expressed in Langerhans cells but are differentially regulated in culture. J Exp Med 1992; 176:1221-6.

34. Trede NS, Geha RS, Chatila T. Transcriptional activation of IL-1β and tumor necrosis factor-α genes by MHC class II ligands. J Immunol 1991; 146:2310-5.

35. Winzen R, Wallach D, Kemper O et al. Selective up-regulation of the 75-kDa tumor necrosis factor (TNF) receptor and its mRNA by TNF and IL-1. J Immunol 1993; 150:4346-53.
36. Kämpgen E, Koch F, Heufler C et al. Understanding the dendritic cell lineage through a study of cytokine receptors. J Exp Med 1994; 179:1767-76.
37. Tang A, Amagai M, Granger LG et al. Adhesion of epidermal Langerhans cells to keratinocytes mediated by E-cadherin. Nature 1993; 361:82-85.
38. Sallusto F, Lanzavecchia A. Efficient presentation of soluble antigen by cultured human dendritic cells is maintained by granulocyte/macrophage colony-stimulating factor plus interleukin 4 and downregulated by tumor necrosis factor α. J Exp Med 1994; 179:1109-18.
39. Gunthert U, Hofmann M, Rudy W et al. A new variant of glycoprotein CD44 confers metastatic potential to rat carcinoma cells. Cell 1991; 65:13-9.
40. Gabrilovich DI, Wood GM, Patterson S et al. Retrovirus-induced immunosuppression via blocking of dendritic cell migration and down-regulation of adhesion molecules. Immunology 1994; 82:82-7.
41. Tabata N, Aiba S, Nakagawa S et al. Sialyl Lewis x, expression on human Langerhans cells. J Invest Dermatol 1993; 101:175-9.
42. Ross EL, Barker JNWN, Allen MH et al. Langerhans cell expression of the selectin ligand, sialyl Lewis x. Immunology 1994; 81:303-8.
43. Le Varlet B, Dezutter-Dambuyant, Staquet MH et al. Human epidermal Langerhans cells express integrins of the β1 subfamily. J Invest Dermatol 1991; 96:518-22.
44. Le Varlet B, Staquet MJ, Dezutter-Dambuyant C et al. In vitro adhesion of human epidermal Langerhans cells to laminin and fibronectin occurs through β1 integrin receptors. J Leukoc Biol 1992; 51:415-20.
45. Aiba S, Nakagawa S, Ozawa H et al. Up-regulation of α4 integrin on activated Langerhans cells: analysis of adhesion molecules on Langerhans cells relating to their migration from skin to draining lymph nodes. J Invest Dermatol 1993; 100:143-7.
46. Ioffreda MD, Whitaker D, Murphy GF. Mast cell degranulation upregulates α6 integrins on epidermal Langerhans cells. J Invest Dermatol 1993; 101:150-4.
47. Halliday GM, Lucas AD. Protein kinase C tranduces the signal for Langerhans cell migration from the epidermis. Immunology 1993; 79:621-6.

ULTRAVIOLET RADIATION-MEDIATED DEFECTS IN LANGERHANS CELL FUNCTION

Paul R. Bergstresser, Akira Takashima

INTRODUCTION: ULTRAVIOLET RADIATION, SKIN, AND LANGERHANS CELLS

ULTRAVIOLET RADIATION AND SKIN

Skin, after exposure to sunlight, exhibits a sequence of predictable changes, including redness (erythema), immediate pigment darkening and tanning, followed later by premature aging and cancer. Although electromagnetic radiation that reaches the earth contains a spectrum of energies, ranging from ultraviolet (UV) to infrared, it is UV radiation in spectrum B (UVB: 290-320 nm) and spectrum A (UVA: 320-400 nm) that are responsible for the majority of these changes. On the other hand, UVA and UVB radiation are unequal in their capacities to affect skin. Specifically, UVB is more efficient in producing erythema and cancer, whereas UVA is the primary cause of immediate pigment darkening and aging.[1]

PHOTOIMMUNOLOGY

Photoimmunology, a relatively new field of investigation, addresses the modulation of immunity by UV radiation. This field, which has developed rapidly over the last 15 years, originated from reports by several investigators that irradiation had the capacity to distort the acquisition of immunity in a fashion that led to tolerance rather than protective immunity (reviewed in ref. 2). This method of inducing tolerance was found to occur for a diverse group of antigens, including contact sensitizers, tumors and nominal antigens. Moreover, there has been considerable interest in the relationship between UV-induced tolerance and carcinogenesis.[3] Although the experiments that defined photoimmunology were conducted in laboratory animals, primarily in mice, there is now sufficient corroborating evidence from other rodent species and from humans to be certain that the effects of irradiation are general rather than limited in scope. The focus of this review is upon mechanisms by which the induction of tolerance is mediated through the activities of Langerhans cells (LC).

T CELL MEDIATED IMMUNITY IN SKIN

The vast majority of studies dealing with UV radiation have addressed its impact on T cell mediated immunity, which depends upon activities of three types of cells: (1) resident *antigen presenting cells* (APC) which, after appropriate stimulation, migrate via lymphatic vessels into regional lymph nodes where they activate immunologically naive T cells—this activation process is achieved most effectively by dendritic cells, which are APC represented in epidermis by LC; (2) specifically activated and highly mobile *T cells* which, after clonal expansion, recirculate preferentially and continuously between lymphoid tissues and peripheral tissues where they survey for the original antigen; (3) *other resident cells*, including keratinocytes, fibroblasts and endothelial cells in skin, which regulate the function of LC through the elaboration of cytokines and the expression of adhesion molecules. Thus, the effects of UV radiation on LC have been detected primarily by examining the emigration of LC and their capacity to activate T cells.

LANGERHANS CELLS

Central to the concept of tissue-specific protective immunity is the knowledge that dendritic cells from various tissues activate T cells that have the capacity to return preferentially to that tissue. As resident epidermal leukocytes of dendritic cell lineage, LC mature into highly effective APC for the activation of immunologically naive T cells, and they have been reported to present several forms of antigens that commonly penetrate or appear in skin, including chemical haptens, microorganisms, alloantigens and tumor-associated antigens (reviewed in ref. 4). More specifically, effective antigen processing and presentation by LC requires a change in their phenotype and function. This requirement for change was first identified when LC were cultured for several days with cytokines known to be produced by keratinocytes. Phenotypic changes in culture include: (1) heightened expression of major histocompatibility complex (MHC) class II molecules, (2) acquired expression of B7-1 and other adhesion molecules [e.g., CD54 (intercellular adhesion molecule 1; ICAM-1) and CD11a/CD18 (lymphocyte function-associated antigen 1; LFA-1)], and (3) decreased expression of E-cadherin. Functional changes in culture include: (1) an increased ability to present peptide antigens to naive T cells, and (2) a reduced capacity to take up and process complex protein antigens. A commonly accepted scenario is that these changes also take place as LC migrate out of the epidermis and into regional lymph nodes.[5]

EPIDERMIS AS A MICROENVIRONMENT

Finally, a recent conceptual advance has been the realization that resident epidermal cells are not independent; rather, as a collective, they establish a functioning "microenvironment."[4] This predicts that LC may not be the only relevant target of irradiation in vivo; keratinocytes have been proposed to serve as "signal transducers" by converting signals triggered by exogenous agents (such as UV radiation) into altered production of cytokines and adhesion molecules.[6]

UVB IRRADIATION IN VIVO: IMPLIED EFFECTS ON THE FUNCTION OF LANGERHANS CELLS

EXPOSURE OF SKIN TO UVB RADIATION

The first experiments to address effects of UV radiation were conducted in vivo, with the limitation that distortions in immune function could be attributed only circumstantially to LC. On the other hand, it soon became apparent that they were quite susceptible to irradiation. We reported in 1980 that surface densities of adenosintriphosphatase (ATPase)-positive LC could be diminished substantially by exposing mice to relatively modest fluences of UV radiation from unfiltered FS sunlamps. As little as 100 J/m² per day delivered on four successive days was sufficient.[7] This capacity of UV radiation to delete LC or to diminish the expression of characteristic cell-surface molecules, such as ATPase and MHC class II antigens, has also been confirmed in humans.[8] Spencer et al[8] have observed that even an ordinary course of treatment with UVB radiation, in fluences sufficient to clear plaque-stage psoriasis, diminishes the number of MHC class II+ LC in volunteer subjects, although the remaining LC tended to express increased levels of class II antigens.

IMMUNIZATION THROUGH UV-IRRADIATED SKIN

Taking advantage of the capacity of UV radiation to decrease surface densities of LC, we subsequently sought to determine whether skin treated in this fashion would retain the capacity to produce contact-sensitivity reactions. Using the reactive hapten dinitrofluorobenzene (DNFB), we observed that application through a site of irradiation failed to induce vigorous immunity.[7] Moreover, this failure at immunization was not a "null event," because mice treated in this fashion would not develop full sensitivity when DNFB was applied a second time, even to previously unirradiated skin. The mice had developed antigen-specific tolerance to a hapten that was first encountered through irradiated skin. This observation was followed by experiments demonstrating that the hapten-specific tolerance could be transferred adoptively with T cells to immunologically naive recipients.[9] Soon thereafter, Elmets et al[10] determined the action spectrum of "low-dose" suppression, observing a peak at 280 nm, and thus differentiating it from the absorption spectra of both DNA and *trans*-urocanic acid (UCA) (see below). These early studies have provided impetus for the development of a "low-dose" or "local" model of UVB-induced immunosuppression.

The defining aspect of what is described above as "low-dose" or "local" immunosuppression was that tolerance would develop only when haptens were painted directly and locally on an irradiated site, and proof of tolerance required a subsequent (unsuccessful) course of conventional immunization. Moreover, the fluences of UV radiation used in these studies did not affect other types of cell-mediated immunity, including graft rejection and the recognition of antigens injected into the dermis. Most importantly, contact sensitivity remained unaffected when haptens were applied to a remote site. Finally, this effect of UV radiation was not limited to mice, as it is now known to occur in humans.[11,12]

From a different perspective, Alcalay and Kripke[13] linked the tolerance produced by low-dose UV radiation to UV-induced carcinogenesis. In their experiments, draining lymph node cells obtained from mice sensitized with DNFB were used as APC. When obtained from mice that were concurrently exposed to a carcinogenic protocol of UV irradiation, their capacity to present DNFB was reduced substantially. Moreover, this reduced activity was present throughout the latent period of tumor development. Thus, the reduced numbers of identifiable LC early in the course of chronic UV irradiation correlated with decreased antigen-presenting activity of LC that drained such sites.

Immunizing Through Unirradiated Skin

In parallel studies, other investigators employed a model with higher fluences of radiation, a model that produced somewhat different results.[3] With higher fluences, the site of irradiation became unimportant; mice became tolerant irrespective of the site of hapten application. Not only did this suggest a different mechanism, it also focused attention away from a direct effect of UV radiation on LC. The implication was that higher amounts of radiation had led to the diffusion of a locally produced factor into the systemic circulation, where it would interfere with the acquisition of immunity in several locations. As will be seen, both *cis*-UCA and interleukin 10 (IL-10) are attractive candidates for this factor. Importantly, immunization after exposure to higher fluences of UV radiation was found to cause suppression for antigens other than contact sensitizers, including nominal antigens and UV-induced tumors. Subsequently, both of these models (low-dose and high-dose) have been used by many investigators. Since recent evidence favors distinct pathogenic mechanisms for these two models,[14] it is important to identify the model that has been employed when attempting to reconcile apparent differences.

Genetic Diversity

Studies with the low-dose model of UV-induced immunosuppression revealed that not all strains of mice were equally susceptible to UV exposure.[15] Even though irradiation depleted ATPase+ LC in all strains of mice, tolerance to DNFB developed only in selected strains. This has suggested that destruction of LC may not be the critical event. Moreover, an intensive search for the relevant genetic factor has implicated polymorphic alleles at two different loci, tumor necrosis factor α (TNF-α) and *lps*.[16] As will be noted below, genetic factors also appear to control susceptibility in humans, and, thus, this model has received considerable attention.[17]

DIRECT EFFECTS OF UV RADIATION ON LANGERHANS CELLS IN VITRO: MECHANISMS FOR UV-INDUCED IMMUNOLOGICAL TOLERANCE

Several lines of evidence have implicated LC as a direct and relevant target of UV irradiation. As noted previously, these were derived from the original observation that LC (or their characteristic markers) could be deleted by relatively modest fluences of radiation. The simplest explanation would be that irradiation kills LC, with sensitization not achieved in their absence;[18] this has the disadvantage of not addressing the mechanism of antigen-specific tolerance. A second mechanism that continues to receive considerable support is that a unique APC population, one that resides ordinarily in the dermis or beyond, immigrates into the epidermis or becomes activated in response to irradiation. This mechanism has the advantage of providing a compelling rationale for the induction of tolerance, and work by Cooper and his associates[19] has provided substantial recent confirmation. Despite its merit in providing a rationale for events in vivo, this mechanism will not be discussed further, because it is beyond the scope of this review. Finally, as implied above, a third mechanism is that LC change their APC potential in response to irradiation. As we focus on that possibility, it should be kept in mind, however, that none of these mechanisms are mutually exclusive.

ANTIGEN PROCESSING

Two relevant events follow antigen uptake and emigration of LC into draining lymph nodes: antigen processing and antigen presentation. Processing itself includes a series of metabolic steps through which complex proteins are cleaved proteolytically into relatively short peptides, which then are selected for their capacity to "fit" into MHC class I or class II molecules. To begin to examine the processing, Girolomoni et al first examined in vitro acidification of endosomal compartments by human LC,[20] observing no obvious acidification defect that could be attributed to irradiation. In retrospect, this should not have been surprising, because it is now apparent that the induction of tolerance also requires effective processing. Thus, to our knowledge there has been no further search for a selective effect of UV radiation on antigen processing itself.

ANTIGEN PRESENTATION

Substantial evidence does document the capacity of irradiation to affect antigen presentation directly. Soon after our report that relatively modest fluences of radiation would distort immunization in vivo, Stingl and his colleagues observed that epidermal cells (including LC) which were irradiated in vitro lost their capacity to present nominal antigens to primed T cells.[21] Using anti-MHC class II antibodies, they had determined that LC were responsible for antigen presentation and, by implication, that irradiation had distorted that function. On the other hand, the use of epidermal cells without purification of LC meant that the identity of the target cell and the photoreceptor could not be addressed. Subsequently, Sauder and his colleagues reported that irradiation of antigen-pulsed epidermal cells (including LC) would lead to antigen-specific tolerance rather than immunity when administered in vivo.[22] Thus, in both sets of experiments, the role of large numbers of accompanying keratinocytes was not evaluated; clarification of their role awaited the development of techniques to isolate LC from other epidermal cells.

Having developed a fluorescence-activated cell sorter (FACS)-based technique for epidermal cell isolation, Sullivan et al went on to observe that only LC among epidermal cells had the capacity to confer unambiguous immunity when hapten-derivatized and infused intravenously.[23] It was also of interest that hapten-derivatized keratinocytes infused in similar numbers had no perceptible effect. In a subsequent study, it was confirmed that isolated LC would induce contact sensitivity when hapten-derivatized and administered intravenously, but, more importantly, demonstrated that when irradiation preceded hapten derivatization, tolerance was induced instead. Within this context, it was also observed that LC administered intravenously would return preferentially to skin and that the returning LC retained the capacity to induce sensitivity or tolerance, depending on their recent experience with UV radiation.[24] Thus, it was concluded that irradiated LC alone were sufficient to induce tolerance in vivo.

PREFERENTIAL ACTIVATION OF T HELPER 2 SUBSET
BY UV-IRRADIATED LANGERHANS CELLS

Several studies conducted in vitro have provided insight into mechanisms by which direct effects of UV radiation lead to tolerance rather than immunity in vivo. In the first, Simon et al[25] observed that highly purified LC lost the capacity to present a complex protein antigen, KLH, effectively to T helper cells of type 1 (Th1 cells) when UV-irradiated. By contrast, their capacity to activate Th2 cells was unaffected by the same fluences of UV radiation. In light of the contemporary concept that Th1 and Th2 subsets play distinct (and competing) immunologic roles in vivo, with Th1 cells being responsible for delayed-type hypersensitivity (reviewed in ref. 26), UV radiation may induce tolerance by causing a selective inability of LC to activate Th1 cells. In the face of preserved Th2 activation, IL-10 derived from Th2 cells would inhibit the activation of Th1 cells, leaving Th2 cells unrestrained.

INDUCTION OF T CELL ANERGY
BY UV-IRRADIATED LANGERHANS CELLS

A second mechanism for the ability of UV irradiation to convert effective immunity into tolerance in vivo emerged from a subsequent study reported by Simon et al.[27] In these studies, Th1 cells were again stimulated with KLH-pulsed and UV-irradiated LC. Not only did irradiation prevent activation, but upon further examination the responder T cells were observed to have become anergic to subsequent stimulation, even by unirradiated LC. Activation had been replaced by anergy. In fact, clonal anergy is now favored as a relevant mechanism for the induction of peripheral tolerance after T cell development, leading to the possibility that irradiation induces tolerance directly by this mechanism. Importantly, clonal anergy has been most commonly induced by nonprofessional APC that do not express all relevant accessory molecules, especially members of the B7 family.[28]

IL-1β

Recent evidence favors an important role for LC-derived IL-1β in the induction of contact sensitivity in skin.[29] We have taken advantage of a recently developed line of dendritic cells derived from mouse epidermis.[30] These dendritic cell lines, termed XS, constitutively express IL-1β mRNA.[31] When XS cells were exposed to UVB radiation, constitutive expression of IL-1β mRNA was downregulated in a dose-dependent fashion, with a significant reduction at 200 J/m². Taken together, these observations suggest that abrogated IL-1β mRNA expression is one mechanism leading to UV-induced impairment of APC function. Notably, UV-induced IL-1β downregulation and impairment of APC function were both prevented by preincubation of XS cells with purified catalase, and both were inducible by brief exposure to exogenous hydrogen peroxide.[32] Thus, the generation of hydrogen peroxide by UVB radiation appears to be essential for at least two of its deleterious effects on dendritic cells in skin.

MATURATIONAL STATES OF LANGERHANS CELLS

Finally, it has been reported recently that UVB susceptibility of LC varies depending on their state of maturation.[33] Focusing on accessory cell function, Tang and Udey observed that UVB radiation prevented upregulation of CD54 during initial LC culture.[34] At the same time, LC became increasingly resistant to effects of irradiation. In other words, relatively immature LC (i.e., freshly isolated LC) were more susceptible to UV radiation than were LC that had already matured in culture. These observations lead to the hypothesis that UV radiation alters antigen-presenting profiles of LC by preventing their maturation into fully professional dendritic cells.

UV RADIATION MODULATES LANGERHANS CELL FUNCTION INDIRECTLY BY AFFECTING NEIGHBORING KERATINOCYTES

A growing literature documents the capacity of UV radiation to alter the expression of adhesion molecules and the production of cytokines by keratinocytes, a major constituent of epidermis. Because of the various roles played by these molecules during cell trafficking and during antigen presentation, distortions in their function remain an attractive possibility for mediating at least some of the deleterious effects of UV radiation. As will be seen, a direct etiologic link between adhesion molecules and altered function has not been identified, but links to cytokine expression are quite compelling.

ADHESION MOLECULES

ICAM-1, with its ligand partner, LFA-1, facilitates the adhesion of T cells to dendritic cells during antigen presentation as well as the trafficking of lymphoid cells. ICAM-1 is normally not expressed on keratinocytes, but it was demonstrated by Norris et al[35] that ICAM-1 expression is triggered and then downregulated in a biphasic fashion by in vitro UV irradiation. Subsequently, Norris et al[36] carried these experiments further by examining the effects of monochromatic (300 nm) radiation on the expression of three adhesion molecules in human skin in vivo: ICAM-1, endothelial leukocyte adhesion molecule 1 (ELAM-1), and vascular cell adhesion molecule 1 (VCAM-1). ELAM-1 on vascular endothelia was upregulated rapidly, peaking at 24 hours, and diminishing thereafter. By contrast, VCAM-1 on endothelial cells and ICAM-1 on keratinocytes were not affected. Although there still exists some conflict, these studies have suggested a unique pathway through which UV radiation indirectly alters LC function; i.e., through regulating the expression of adhesion molecules by keratinocytes and other cell types in skin.

CYTOKINES

For more than a decade, it has been known that UV radiation has the capacity to upregulate cytokine production by epidermal keratinocytes. On the other hand, there appears to be very little specificity in this effect, as the list is quite lengthy: IL-1,[37] TNF-α,[38] IL-10,[39] granulocyte/macrophage colony-stimulating factor (GM-CSF),[40] and IL-3.[40] Moreover, irradiation also upregulates the production of antagonists of IL-1, including contra-IL-1 and the IL-1 receptor antagonist, which have been proposed as relevant mediators of immunosuppression in skin.[41,42] It is likely that this list will grow ever longer as novel cytokines and novel mechanisms of regulation are uncovered. In the meantime, two lines of investigation have provided compelling evidence that UV-induced upregulation of TNF-α and IL-10 are both relevant.

IL-10

Rivas and Ullrich reported in 1992 that IL-10 was released by keratinocytes that were irradiated in vitro. Moreover, when introduced parenterally, keratinocyte-derived IL-10 had the capacity to interrupt immunization, leading to tolerance instead.[39] Relevance of this mechanism to in vivo irradiation was then supplied by the subsequent experiment in which parenterally administered antibodies against IL-10 interrupted the development of tolerance in the high-dose UV-irradiation model. This revealing work has been complemented by recent reports from Enk et al, indicating that IL-10 also has the capacity to inhibit antigen presentation by LC in vitro, in a fashion that leads to clonal anergy in Th1 cells.[43] Thus, IL-10, most likely produced by UV-irradiated keratinocytes, remains a prominent candidate for mediating effects of UV irradiation in vivo. On the other hand, the source of IL-10 may not yet be certain, because recent evidence from Cooper and his associates indicates that, in humans, infiltrating macrophages are a more significant source of IL-10 than are keratinocytes.[44]

TNF-α

Streilein and colleagues have provided strong support for the relevance of TNF-α produced by keratinocytes to the capacity of UV radiation to cause immunosuppression. This work began with the knowledge that "low-dose" UV radiation would prevent the induction of contact sensitivity to DNFB.[7] It also relied on the knowledge cited previously that one of the genes determining UV susceptibility is in the TNF-α locus. It was proposed that TNF-α ultimately interrupts the induction of contact sensitivity by preventing epidermal LC from carrying hapten into draining lymph nodes. More specifically, they observed that TNF-α, when injected intradermally into a site of ear challenge, would enhance expression of contact sensitivity to DNFB. Interestingly, TNF-α amplified the expression of contact sensitivity in the ears of all mouse strains, but anti-TNF-α antibodies neutralized UVB-enhanced contact sensitivity only in UVB-susceptible mice. These findings support the proposition that TNF-α, released from UVB-exposed epidermal cells, is a critical mediator of the effects of UVB radiation on both the induction and the elicitation of contact sensitivity (reviewed in ref. 16). On the other hand, Moodycliffe et al[45] have observed that UVB enhances migration of LC to regional lymph nodes. Thus, it appears that further studies are required to determine the role played by TNF-α in UV-induced modulation of cutaneous immunity.

INTERPRETING ACTION SPECTRA OF UV-INDUCED IMMUNOSUPPRESSION: ROLES PLAYED BY UROCANIC ACID

For radiation to become biologically relevant, it first must be absorbed by a chromophore in the target tissue. Chromophores of immunologic interest have included DNA, *trans*-UCA, and cyclic amino acids and unsaturated lipids at the cell surface. When a chromophore absorbs radiation of an appropriate wavelength, it is activated to a higher energy state, a process that often confers chemical reactivity. Depending on the nature of the reactivity, the duration of the activated state, and the location of the chromophore, cellular metabolic pathways may be altered substantially. Ultimately, the effect of photon absorption may be beneficial, as in vitamin D synthesis, trivial, as occurs when melanin is the photoreceptor, or destructive, as with the generation of cyclobutane-pyrimidine dimers in DNA or reactive oxygen species at the surfaces of cells (see below).

Critical to the following analysis, each biological molecule has a characteristic absorption spectrum, which reflects the efficiency for absorption of electromagnetic energy at various wavelengths. Thus, UV-radiation effects in skin are mediated by molecules that efficiently absorb the UV spectrum. This means that the effects of radiation within a tissue are mediated more efficiently by some wavelengths than by others; this efficiency is termed the action spectrum (reviewed in ref. 46). In fact, the action spectrum for an effect can be determined experimentally by exposing cells to radiation of various wavelengths and then measuring its effects, such as thymine-dimer formation, cell death or redness in skin. Action spectra have even been used to identify photoreceptors, because under ideal conditions, they should be similar to the absorption spectra of relevant molecules. Thus, by matching action spectra with absorption spectra, candidate molecules can be determined. This method of empiric analysis is most accurate when a single and highly absorbent molecule alone is responsible for a highly specific effect. Moreover, it is also most accurate when experiments are conducted in vitro and without an interposed epidermis or stratum corneum.

A revealing set of experiments in which an in vivo action spectrum identified a candidate molecule was reported in a series of papers by Noonan and DeFabo.[47] They reported that the action spectrum for the development of systemic immunosuppression (tolerance) for a contact sensitizer in mice was similar to the absorption spectrum of a previously underappreciated molecule that occurs in high concentrations in skin, *trans*-UCA.[48] Importantly, UV absorption by *trans*-UCA leads to an unstable molecular state followed by conversion to a different isomer, *cis*-UCA. Because of a simultaneous change in solubility, isomerization leads to diffusion throughout skin and into the systemic circulation. Interestingly, also, *cis*-UCA has been found to be immunosuppressive. These observations have led to an array of reports concerning the effectiveness of *cis*-UCA in interrupting immunization, particularly with respect to viral antigens.[49]

Work with UCA has also opened a new area of research in photoimmunology. Knowing that UCA is a metabolite of the amino acid L-histidine, Reilly and DeFabo[50] reasoned that increased dietary histidine might raise levels of UCA in the skin, in turn enhancing UV-induced suppression of contact sensitivity. In fact, this hypothesis turned out to be correct. Mice given a histidine-rich diet did develop increased levels of UCA; moreover, the degree of UV-induced suppression of contact sensitivity increased proportionately. Not only do these findings provide additional circumstantial support for the relevance of *trans*-UCA in the generation of tolerance, they also provide evidence that a dietary element, L-histidine, (although provided in relatively high amounts) would enhance UV-induced immune suppression in the high-dose model.

Although *trans*-UCA has not been established as the only relevant photoreceptor in UV-induced suppression, it is quite certain that the product of photoconversion, *cis*-UCA, is highly active in producing immunosuppression in vivo. Moreover, several mechanisms of action for this effect have been considered in recent studies, including competition with histamine as an immunomodulatory factor,[51] and stimulation of TNF-α production, leading to the retention of LC within the epidermis.[16] On the other hand, this is not to say that agreement on the role of UCA is universal; Moodycliffe et al[45] have observed that UVB enhances the migration of LC to regional lymph nodes, whereas *cis*-UCA does not alter migration. Moreover, they observed that narrow-band UVB (311 nm) does cause the isomerization of *trans*-UCA to *cis*-UCA, but that it does not cause immunosuppression.[45] Because *cis*-UCA is formed with either broad-band or 311 nm radiation, and suppression occurs only with broad band, they concluded that *trans*-UCA could not be the photoreceptor. Obviously, further studies will be required to determine the extent to which *cis*-UCA accounts for the UV-induced immunological tolerance.

MOLECULAR MECHANISMS BY WHICH
UV RADIATION ALTERS CELLULAR FUNCTION

DNA

The first and most logical choice among candidate photoreceptors for UV-induced immunosuppression has been DNA. Not
only does DNA absorb radiation within relevant portions of the
UV spectrum, the concept that defects in gene utilization might
lead to altered cellular function is compelling. Kripke and her colleagues[52] conducted studies with the opossum *Monodelphis
domestica*, a marsupial species that resembles humans in its capacity to repair UV-induced pyrimidine-dimer formation when irradiation is followed by exposure to high fluences of visible light;
this process is termed photoreactivation. In their experiments, exposure of UV-irradiated skin subsequent to visible light prevented
the development of immunosuppression in the "high-dose" model.
The simplest interpretation was that cyclobutane-pyrimidine dimer
formation was required for the development of immunosuppression, meaning that DNA was the relevant photoreceptor.

Additional confirmatory evidence for DNA as a relevant photoreceptor came from subsequent studies in which DNA was re-
paired by a different mechanism.[53] Mice were first exposed to UV
radiation and then treated topically with liposomes that contained
a bacterial dimer-specific excision-repair enzyme. Not only did this
treatment decrease the number of pyrimidine dimers in the irradiated epidermis, it also prevented the suppression of both contact
sensitivity to reactive haptens and delayed-type hypersensitivity to
complex proteins. Because of the specificity of this enzyme, the
most logical conclusion was that repair of DNA had prevented
the development of suppression, meaning, once again, that DNA
was the relevant photoreceptor for UV radiation-induced systemic
immunosuppression. Taken together, these studies suggest strongly
that the primary molecular event mediating this type of immunosuppression is the formation of pyrimidine dimers.

CELL MEMBRANES

A third hypothesis, one that has as yet received only modest
attention, concerns the role of unsaturated lipids or tryptophane-
containing proteins within cell membranes. Rationale for this possibility begins with knowledge that the cell surface contains an

array of regulatory molecules that are dependent upon the integrity of their local "environment." Critical to this line of investigation is the regulation of immediate early genes (IEG). IEG are specific genes induced rapidly in response to receptor occupancy; genes in the *jun/fos* and the *egr* families have been studied most extensively.[54,55] A widely accepted model of IEG participation in the normal signaling cascade is as follows: (1) receptor ligation, (2) signal transduction and amplification through second messengers, (3) induction of IEG transcription and translation and (4) binding of IEG products to promoter regions of functional genes which encode the proteins responsible for regulated cell function. Thus, products of IEG serve as nuclear mediators that transduce signals occurring at the plasma membrane to the nuclei.

It has been established by Karin and colleagues that an IEG cascade is activated by UV radiation, although the most comprehensive work employed fibroblasts and radiation in the short wavelength range (UVC). Irradiation of fibroblasts with UVC induces a rapid activation of *c-jun*, *c-fos*, and NFκB.[56] Significantly, UV-dependent activation of NFκB occurs in cells without nuclei, indicating that the initial event occurs at or near the plasma membrane and not in the nucleus.[56] Supporting the idea of interference with the normal signaling cascade, Ha-ras, Src tyrosine kinases and JNK1, a serine/threonine kinase, have been identified as mediators of UV-dependent *c-jun* activation.[57,58] It is also of note that reactive oxygen intermediates play causative roles in UVB-dependent IEG activation.[59]

More recently, UV-dependent IEG activation has been studied in keratinocytes. These studies have revealed that: (1) UVB radiation induces the activation of NFκB in a DNA-independent fashion in A431 keratinocytes,[60] (2) exposure of normal human keratinocytes to solar-simulating irradiation upregulates *c-fos* and downregulates *c-myc* mRNA expression,[61] and (3) exposure of human skin to solar-simulating radiation induces *c-fos* mRNA expression in epidermis.[62] In our own experiments, A431 keratinocytes were exposed to UVB or UVA radiation at different fluences and then examined 60 minutes later for mRNA expression of a panel of IEG. UVB radiation induced a marked upregulation in *c-jun* mRNA, with significant elevation occurring at 25 J/m^2. By contrast, UVA radiation caused minimal upregulation of this gene, even at large fluences (up to 20,000 J/m^2). On the other hand, *fra-1*, a member of the *fos* family, was upregulated by UVA radiation in a dose-dependent fashion, but it was downregulated by UVB radiation. Likewise, *c-myc* was upregulated by UVA and down-regulated by UVB radiation. These results indicate that UVB and UVA activate (and repress) different sets of IEG in a transformed keratinocyte line. Moreover, treatment with superoxide dismutase prevented UVB radiation from triggering *c-jun* upregulation or *c-myc* downregulation, leading to the conclusion that reactive oxygen species may play an essential role in these signaling pathways.[63]

FUTURE PERSPECTIVES

RELEVANCE OF PHOTOIMMUNOLOGY TO HUMAN CARCINOGENESIS

Two groups of investigators have extended to humans the studies conducted previously in rodents, although they do not implicate LC directly. Working with normal control subjects and with patients who have had keratinocyte-derived skin cancers, Yoshikawa et al[11] observed that nearly 50% of the normal subjects developed tolerance when immunized through irradiated skin. By contrast, virtually 100% of patients who had a history of skin cancer became tolerant, suggesting that UV susceptibility was a significant risk factor for UV-induced cancer development. These investigators then examined additional subjects for the phenotypic trait of UV susceptibility, confirming that it was relatively high in Caucasians (approx. 40-45%). On the other hand, this incidence was equally high in individuals with deeply pigmented skin, who have a low incidence of skin cancer.[64] Thus, UV susceptibility is one, but not the only, risk factor for the development of skin cancer.

In other studies, Cooper et al[12] examined the dose responsiveness for UV susceptibility. When UV radiation sufficient to induce redness (the minimal erythemal dose or MED) was administered prior to hapten painting with dinitrochlorobenzene (DNCB), they observed a dose-related reduction in the degree of sensitization. Even with doses below the MED, they observed a decreased frequency of strongly positive responses. Fully 31% of subjects who were immunized initially through skin receiving erythemogenic doses of UV became tolerant. Monitoring APC in the epidermis revealed that erythemogenic regimens induced the appearance of CD1a⁻, HLA-DR⁺ macrophages and depleted resident LC. They concluded that even subclinical doses of UV radiation had a significant modulatory effect on the ability of humans to generate a T cell-mediated response to antigens introduced through irradiated skin.

IS IMMUNOSUPPRESSION PREVENTABLE WITH SUNSCREENS?

An important argument has developed concerning whether commercial sunscreens that prevent sunlight-induced erythema are able to prevent immunosuppression as well. In 1981, Gurish et al,[65] using unfiltered FS sunlamps in a systemic suppression model (relatively high fluence of UVB radiation and a contact sensitizer applied to unirradiated skin), reported that a para-amino benzoic acid (PABA)-containing sunscreen failed to prevent the development of immunosuppression, even though obvious damage to skin had apparently been prevented. By contrast, Morison reported some time later that the same chemical, PABA, did prevent immunosuppression.[66] Later, Fisher et al[67] reported that a sunscreen containing Padimate O and oxybenzone was totally incapable of preventing the immunologic suppression of contact hypersensitivity. Finally, Reeve et al[68] reported that a sunscreen containing octyl-N-dimethyl-p-aminobenzoate did not prevent the development of immunosuppression, whereas 2-ethyl-hexyl-p-methoxycinnamate did. It was instructive that both sunscreens were effective in preventing UV-induced erythema and edema. Some of the controversy among these studies may reflect differences in the light sources, animal species, and/or other experimental components. Because the ultimate goal of photoimmunology research is to prevent (and even reverse) the deleterious effect of solar radiation on cutaneous immunity, it is critical to determine whether commercially available sunscreens can prevent the onset of UV-induced immunosuppression and skin cancer in humans.

REFERENCES

1. Shea CR, Parrish JA. Nonionizing Radiation and the Skin. In: Goldsmith LA, ed. Physiology, Biochemistry, and Molecular Biology of the Skin. New York, Oxford: Oxford University Press, 1991:910-27.
2. Cruz Jr PD, Bergstresser PR. The influence of ultraviolet radiation and other physical and chemical agents on epidermal Langerhans cells. In: Schuler G, ed. Epidermal Langerhans Cells. Boca Raton: CRC Press, 1993:253-71.
3. Kripke ML. Immunology and photocarcinogenesis. J Am Acad Dermatol 1986; 14:149-55.
4. Stingl G, Hauser C, Wolff K. The epidermis: an immunologic microenvironment. In: Fitzpatrick TB, ed. Dermatology in General Medicine. New York: McGraw Hill and Co., 1993:172-97.

5. Aiba S, Nakagawa S, Ozawa H et al. Up-regulation of 4 integrin on activated Langerhans cells: analysis of adhesion molecules on Langerhans cells relating to their migration from skin to draining lymph nodes. J Invest Dermatol 1993; 100:143-7.

6. Barker JN, Mitra RS, Griffiths CE et al. Keratinocytes as initiators of inflammation. Lancet 1991; 337:211-4.

7. Toews GB, Bergstresser PR, Streilein JW. Epidermal Langerhans cell density determines whether contact hypersensitivity or unresponsiveness follows skin painting with DNFB. J Immunol 1980; 134:445-53.

8. Spencer M-J, Vestey JP, Tidman MJ et al. Major histocompatibility class II antigen expression on the surface of epidermal cells from normal and ultraviolet B irradiated subjects. J Invest Dermatol 1993; 100:16-22.

9. Elmets CA, Bergstresser PR, Tigelaar RE et al. Analysis of the mechanism of unresponsiveness produced by haptens painted on skin exposed to low dose ultraviolet radiation. J Exp Med 1983; 158:781-94.

10. Elmets CA, LeVine MJ, Bickers DR. Action spectrum studies for induction of immunologic unresponsiveness to dinitrobenzene following in vivo low dose ultraviolet radiation. Photochem Photobiol 1985; 42:391-7.

11. Yoshikawa T, Rae V, Bruins-Slot W et al. Susceptibility to effects of UVB radiation on induction of contact hypersensitivity as a risk factor for skin cancer in humans. J Invest Dermatol 1990; 95:530-6.

12. Cooper KD, Oberhelman L, Hamilton TA et al. UV exposure reduces immunization rates and promotes tolerance to epicutaneous antigens in humans: relationship to dose, CD1a⁻ DR⁺ epidermal macrophage induction, and Langerhans cell depletion. Proc Natl Acad Sci USA 1992; 89:8497-8501.

13. Alcalay J, Kripke ML. Antigen-presenting activity of draining lymph node cells from mice painted with a contact allergen during ultraviolet carcinogenesis. J Immunol 1991; 146:1717-21.

14. Wolf P, Donawho CK, Kripke ML. Analysis of the protective effect of different sunscreens on ultraviolet radiation-induced local and systemic suppression of contact hypersensitivity and inflammatory responses in mice. J Invest Dermatol 1993; 100:254-9.

15. Streilein JW, Bergstresser PR. Genetic basis of ultraviolet B effects on contact hypersensitivity. Immunogenetics 1988; 27:252-8.

16. Streilein JW. Sunlight and skin-associated lymphoid tissues (SALT): If UVB is the trigger and TNF is its mediator, what is the message? J Invest Dermatol 1993; 100:47S-52S.

17. Vincek V, Kurimoto I, Medema JP et al. Tumor necrosis factor α polymorphism correlates with deleterious effects of ultraviolet B light on cutaneous immunity. Cancer Res 1993; 53:728-32.

18. Tang A, Udey MC. Doses of ultraviolet radiation that modulate accessory cell activity and ICAM-1 expression are ultimately cytotoxic for murine epidermal Langerhans cells. J Invest Dermatol 1992; 99:71S-73S.

19. Hammerberg C, Duraiswamy N, Cooper KD. Active induction of unresponsiveness (tolerance) to DNFB by in vivo ultraviolet-exposed epidermal cells is dependent upon infiltrating class II MHC+ CD11b bright (superscript) monocyte/macrophagic cells. J Immunol 1994; 153:4915-24.

20. Girolomoni G, Cruz Jr PD, Bergstresser PR. Internalization and acidification of surface HLA-DR molecules by epidermal Langerhans cells: A paradigm for antigen processing. J Invest Dermatol 1990; 94:753-60.

21. Stingl G, Gazze-Stingl LA, Aberer W et al. Antigen presentation by murine epidermal Langerhans cells and its alteration by UVB light. J Immunol 1981; 127:1707-13.

22. Sauder DN, Tamaki K, Moshell AN et al. Introduction of tolerance to topically applied TNCB using TNP-conjugated ultraviolet light-irradiated epidermal cells. J Immunol 1981; 127:261-6.

23. Sullivan S, Bergstresser PR, Tigelaar RE et al. Induction and regulation of contact hypersensitivity by resident, bone marrow-derived, dendritic epidermal cells: Langerhans cells and Thy-1+ epidermal cells. J Immunol 1986; 137:2460-7.

24. Cruz Jr PD, Tigelaar RE, Bergstresser PR. Langerhans cells that migrate to skin after intravenous infusion regulate the induction of contact hypersensitivity. J Immunol 1990; 144:2486-92.

25. Simon JC, Cruz PD, Bergstresser PR et al. Low dose ultraviolet B-irradiated Langerhans cells preferentially activate CD4+ cells of the T helper 2 subset. J Immunol 1990; 145:2087-91.

26. Mosmann TR, Schumacher JH, Street NE et al. Diversity of cytokine synthesis and function of mouse CD4+ T cells. Immunol Rev 1991; 123:209-29.

27. Simon JC, Tigelaar RE, Bergstresser PR et al. UVB radiation converts Langerhans cells from immunogenic to tolerogenic antigen presenting cells. Induction of specific clonal anergy in CD4+ T helper 1 cells. J Immunol 1991; 146:485-91.

28. Gimmi CD, Freeman GJ, Gribben JG et al. Human T-cell clonal anergy is induced by antigen presentation in the absence of B7 costimulation. Proc Natl Acad Sci USA 1993; 90:6586-90.

29. Enk AH, Angeloni VL, Udey MC et al. An essential role for Langerhans cell-derived IL-1β in the initiation of primary immune responses in skin. J Immunol 1993; 150:3698-704.

30. Xu S, Ariizumi K, Caceres-Dittmar G et al. Successive generation of antigen-presenting, dendritic cell lines from murine epidermis. J Immunol 1994; 154:2697-705.

31. Xu S, Ariizumi K, Edelbaum D et al. Cytokine-dependent regulation of growth and maturation in murine epidermal dendritic cell lines. Eur J Immunol 1995; in press.

32. Caceres-Dittmar G, Ariizumi K, Xu S et al. Hydrogen peroxide mediates UVB-induced impairment of antigen presentation and downregulation of IL-1β mRNA expression in a murine epidermal-derived dendritic cell line. Photochem Photobiol 1995; in press.

33. Tang A, Udey MC. Differential sensitivity of freshly isolated and cultured murine Langerhans cells to ultraviolet B radiation and chemical fixation. Eur J Immunol 1992; 22:581-6.

34. Tang A, Udey MC. Effects of ultraviolet radiation on murine epidermal Langerhans cells: doses of ultraviolet radiation that modulate ICAM-1 (CD54) expression and inhibit Langerhans cell function cause delayed cytotoxicity in vitro. J Invest Dermatol 1992; 99:83-9.

35. Norris DA, Lyons MD, Middleton MH et al. Ultraviolet radiation can either suppress or induce expression of intercellular adhesion molecule 1 (ICAM-1) on the surface of cultured human keratinocytes. J Invest Dermatol 1990; 95:132-8.

36. Norris P, Poston RN, Thomas DS et al. The expression of endothelial leukocyte adhesion molecule-1 (ELAM-1), intercellular adhesion molecule-1 (ICAM-1),and vascular cell adhesion molecule-1 (VCAM-1) in experimental cutaneous inflammation: a comparison of ultraviolet B erythema and delayed hypersensitivity. J Invest Dermatol 1991; 96:763-70.

37. Kupper TS, Chua AO, Flood P et al. Interleukin 1 gene expression in cultured human keratinocytes is augmented by ultraviolet irradiation. J Clin Invest 1987; 80:430-6.

38. Kock A, Schwarz T, Kirnbauer R et al. Human keratinocytes are a source for tumor necrosis factor : evidence for synthesis and release upon stimulation with endotoxin or ultraviolet light. J Exp Med 1990; 172:1609-14.

39. Riva JM, Ullrich SE. Systemic suppression of delayed-type hypersensitivity by supernatants from UV-irradiated keratinocytes. An essential role for keratinocyte-derived IL-10. J Immunol 1992; 149:3865-71.

40. Gallo RL, Staszewski R, Sauder DN et al. Regulation of GM-CSF and IL-3 production from the murine keratinocyte cell line PAM 212 following exposure to ultraviolet radiation. J Invest Dermatol 1991; 97:203-9(abstract).

41. Krutmann J, Schwarz T, Kirnbauer R et al. Epidermal cell-contra-interleukin 1 inhibits human accessory function by specifically blocking interleukin 1 activity. Photochem Photobiol 1990; 52:783-8.

42. Schwarz T, Urbanska A, Gschnait F et al. UV-irradiated epidermal cells produce a specific inhibitor of interleukin 1 activity. J Immunol 1987; 138:1457-63.

43. Enk AH, Angeloni VL, Udey MC et al. Inhibition of Langerhans cell antigen-presenting function by IL-10. A role for IL-10 in induction of tolerance. J Immunol 1993; 151:2390-8.

44. Kang K, Hammberberg C, Meunier L et al. CD11b+ macrophages that infiltrate human epidermis after in vivo ultraviolet exposure potently produce IL-10 and represent the major secretory source of epidermal IL-10 protein. J Immunol 1994; 153:5256-64.

45. Moodycliffe AM, Kimber I, Norval M. The effect of ultraviolet B irradiation and urocanic acid isomers on dendritic cell migration. Immunology 1992; 77:394-9.

46. Coohill TP. Photobiology School. Action spectra again? Photochem Photobiol 1991; 54:859-70.

47. Noonan FP, DeFabo EC. Immunosuppression by ultraviolet B radiation: initiation by urocanic acid. Immunol Today 1992; 13:250-4.

48. DeFabo EC, Noonan FP. Mechanism of immune suppression by ultraviolet irradiation in vivo: evidence for the existence of a unique photoreceptor in skin and its role in photoimmunology. J Exp Med 1983; 157:84-98.

49. Norval M, Simpson TJ, Bardshiri E et al. Urocanic acid analogues and the suppression of the delayed type hypersensitivity response to Herpes simplex virus. Photochem Photobiol 1989; 49:633-9.

50. Reilly SK, DeFabo EC. Dietary histidine increases mouse skin urocanic acid levels and enhances UV-induced immune suppression of contact hypersensitivity. Photochem Photobiol 1991; 53:431-8.

51. Norval M, Gilmour JW, Simpson TJ. The effect of histamine receptor antagonists on immunosuppression induced by the cis-isomer of urocanic acid. Photodermatol Photoimmunol Photomed 1990; 7:243-8.

52. Applegate LA, Ley RD, Alcalay J et al. Identification of the molecular target for the suppression of contact hypersensitivity by ultraviolet radiation. J Exp Med 1989; 170:1117-31.

53. Kripke ML, Cox PA, Lori GA et al. Pyrimidine dimers in the DNA initiate systemic immunosuppression in UV-irradiated mice. Proc Natl Acad Sci USA 1992; 89:7516-29.

54. Angel P, Karin M. The role of Jun, Fos, and the AP-1 complex in cell-proliferation and transformation. Biochem Biophys Acta 1991; 1072:129-57.

55. Sukhatme VP. The Egr transcription factor family: From signal transduction to kidney differentiation. Kidney International 1992; 41:550-3.

56. Devary Y, Rosett C, DiDonato JA et al. NF-kappa B activation by ultraviolet light not dependent on a nuclear signal. Science 1993; 261:1442-5.

57. Devary Y, Engelberg D, Klein C et al. The UV response involving the Ras signaling pathway and AP-1 transcription factors is conserved between yeast and mammals. Cell 1994; 77:381-90.

58. Derijard B, Hibi M, Wu IH et al. JNK1: a protein kinase stimulated by UV light and Ha-Ras that binds and phosphorylates the c-Jun activation domain. Cell 1994; 76:1025-37.

59. Devary Y, Gottlieb RA, Smeal T et al. The mammalian ultraviolet response is triggered by activation of Src tyrosine kinases. Cell 1992; 71:1081-91.

60. Simon MM, Aragane Y, Schwarz A et al. UVB light induces nuclear factor B (NFκB) activity independently from chromosomal DNA damage in cell-free cytosolic extracts. J Invest Dermatol 1994; 102:422-7.

61. Garmyn M, Yaar M, Boileau N et al. Effect of aging and habitual sun exposure on the genetic response of cultured human keratinocytes to solar-simulated irradiation. J Invest Dermatol 1992; 99:743-8.

62. Roddy PK, Garmyn M, Park H-Y et al. Ultraviolet irradiation induces c-fos but not c-Ha-ras proto-oncogene expression in human epidermis. J Invest Dermatol 1994; 102:296-9.
63. Ariizumi K, Bergstresser PR, Takashima A. Wavelength-specific induction of immediate early genes by ultraviolet radiation. Photochem Photobiol 1995; submitted.
64. Vermeer M, Schmieder GJ, Yoshikawa T et al. Effects of ultraviolet B light on cutaneous immune responses of humans with deeply pigmented skin. J Invest Dermatol 1991; 97:729-34.
65. Gurish MF, Roberts LK, Krueger GG et al. The effect of various sunscreen agents on skin damage and the induction of tumor susceptibility in mice subjected to ultraviolet irradiation. J Invest Dermatol 1981; 76:246-51.
66. Morison WL. The effect of a sunscreen containing para-aminobenzoic acid on the systemic immunologic alterations induced in mice by exposure to UVB radiation. J Invest Dermatol 1984; 83:405-8.
67. Fisher MS, Menter JM, Willis I. Ultraviolet radiation-induced suppression of contact hypersensitivity in relation to padimate O and oxybenzone. J Invest Dermatol 1989; 92:337-41.
68. Reeve VE, Bosnic M, Boehm-Wilcox C et al. Differential protection by two sunscreens from UV radiation-induced immunosuppression. J Invest Dermatol 1991; 97:624-8.

CHAPTER 9

PRESENTATION OF TUMOR ANTIGENS BY LANGERHANS CELLS AND OTHER DENDRITIC CELLS

Stephan Grabbe, Richard D. Granstein

INTRODUCTION: DOES IT MAKE SENSE TO STUDY TUMOR ANTIGEN PRESENTATION?

It has long been disputed whether human or animal tumors carry immunogenic epitopes on their surface that allow for recognition and destruction of tumor cells by the host's immune system. Whereas earlier studies concluded that experimentally induced tumors are often immunogenic, while spontaneously arising neoplasms lack antigenic epitopes, it is now generally accepted that many spontaneously arising malignancies also carry immunogenic epitopes on their cell surfaces. In the clinical situation, the immunogenicity of some tumors—especially in the case of melanoma—is evident by their infiltration with leukocytes as well as by the phenomenon of spontaneous partial or complete tumor regression. In vitro, tumor-specific cytotoxic T lymphocyte (CTL) activity and cytokine secretion of T cells after coculture with tumor targets has been shown for human primary and metastatic melanoma, and both CD4+ and CD8+ tumor-infiltrating lymphocytes have been

The Immune Functions of Epidermal Langerhans Cells, edited by Heidrun Moll.
© 1995 R.G. Landes Company.

cloned.[1,2] Furthermore, the exact peptide sequences of some of these melanoma antigens are known (Table 9.1).[3,4] Thus, at least with regard to some cutaneous neoplasms, there is formal proof that they can be immunostimulatory.

Tumors are capable of inducing a wide variety of immunological reactions within their hosts. Factors influencing the type of the immune response generated include the individual tumor type, the immune status of the host, the mechanism of tumor induction, the organ and the microenvironment in which it arises. With regard to chemically and ultraviolet (UV) radiation-induced tumors of the skin, the existence of tumor epitopes that induce protective, CD4- or CD8-mediated tumor immunity, as well as of those that result in the formation of suppressor T cells (T_S), has been demonstrated.[5-7] Since all antigen-specific immune responses require antigen presentation, the generation of tumor-specific immunity should also involve the action of antigen-presenting cells (APC). By logical deduction, several conditions must be fulfilled for the establishment of tumor immunity: (1) tumor-specific antigen(s) must be present on the surface of malignant cells; (2) APC must be present in the vicinity of the tumors that are able to acquire, potentially process and present the antigen(s) in the context of major histocompatibility complex (MHC) class I or class II molecules; (3) antigen-carrying APC must establish contact with naive T cells and be able to sensitize them to tumor-associated

Table 9.1. Peptide sequences derived from human melanoma that stimulate autologous CTL*

Gene/Protein	Sequences
MAGE-1	EADPTGHSY
	SAYGEPRKL
MAGE-3	EVDPIGHLY
Tyrosinase	MLLAVLYCL
	YMNGTMSQV
pMel-17	YLEPGPVTA
	LLDGTATLRL
MART-1/Melan-A	AAGIGILTV

* adapted from Slingluff CL et al, Curr Opin Immunol 1994; 6:733-40.

antigens (TAA); (4) antigen-carrying APC must also be able to elicit effector T cell responses that ultimately lead to the destruction of the tumor cells; (5) regulatory mechanisms must exist that control the type, extent and duration of the immune response.

Antigen presentation is a complex process with special requirements both for the APC as well as for the T cell type the antigen is presented to. Within the past decade, the central role of dendritic cells as APC for the induction of primary immune responses has clearly been demonstrated.[8] The conditions required for sensitization of naive hosts ("unprimed system") differ from those necessary to elicit a secondary immune response in primed systems. Whereas various cell types readily present antigen to primed T cells (macrophages, activated B and T cells, endothelial cells, fibroblasts, keratinocytes, etc.), only dendritic APC are believed to have the capacity to sensitize naive, unprimed T cells.[8,9] Thus, it appears logical to speculate that dendritic APC are critically involved in induction and perhaps also in elicitation of tumor-immune responses. Since Langerhans cells (LC) are the principal APC of the epidermis, the recognition and presentation of TAA by LC may be a prerequisite for the establishment of specific immunity against cutaneous neoplasms. This review summarizes the role of LC in tumor immunity and the effects of some cytokines and tumors themselves on tumor-antigen presentation by dendritic APC, and attempts to evaluate the potential use of dendritic APC for tumor immunotherapy.

THE IMMUNE-SURVEILLANCE CONCEPT

The finding that an alteration of the immune status of the host results in increased tumor growth and incidence (e.g., in the case of renal transplant patients) implies that there are at least some connections between the immune system and the outgrowth of neoplasms, and suggests that immunological defense mechanisms against newly emerging tumors may exist. Whereas convincing evidence for the existence of tumor-immune surveillance mechanisms *in general* is still lacking, there is evidence that immune surveillance mechanisms against emerging tumors may indeed exist *within the skin*. This view is supported by several lines of evidence: (1) Immunosuppressed patients have a vastly increased incidence of cutaneous neoplasms within sun-exposed areas, but—with the exception of lymphomas and a few other, mostly virally induced tumors—not of other malignancies (reviewed in ref. 10). Tumor incidence increases with the degree of immunosuppression and cumulative dose of UV-radiation exposure, strongly suggesting a correlation between the degree of immunocompetence and skin-cancer formation. Moreover, skin-cancer patients may have an increased sensitivity to UV radiation-induced suppression of contact hypersensitivity, compared to age-matched controls without skin cancer,[11] providing experimental evidence that immune-surveillance mechanisms are present in normal human skin. (2) Individuals with genetic disorders associated with decreased cellular immunocompetence may also have higher incidence of skin tumors. (3) UV irradiation in mice is accompanied by specific alterations of the immune response in these animals, which are critical for tumor formation since UV-induced skin tumors are often highly antigenic and would be immunologically rejected in normal animals, but grow progressively in UV-irradiated mice (reviewed in refs. 10, 12). (4) In mice, resistance to tumor induction decreases with age in a fashion similar to general immune reactivity decline, suggesting that mice lose with age the capacity to mount immune responses that control tumor growth.[13] (5) Several studies have demonstrated that cutaneous APC have the capacity to recognize TAA and to induce protective tumor immunity in naive mice as well as to elicit T cell mediated, MHC-restricted tumor-specific effector-cell responses in vivo and in vitro, leading to tumor-cell destruction (discussed in detail below). Thus, several lines of evidence confirm an interaction between growing tumors and the host's immune system, at least within the skin.

However, the progressive growth of tumors carrying immunogenic epitopes in an immunocompetent host, despite obvious immune recognition in situ and immune reactivity in vitro, represents a striking paradox in tumor immunology. A possible hypothesis to explain this phenomenon is that immune-surveillance mechanisms exist within the skin which detect and eliminate immunogenic neoplasms before they become clinically apparent, and that only tumors resistant to immunological attack are able to grow progressively under normal conditions in situ. In this concept, carcinogens, which often also inhibit tumor immune recognition, may overwhelm immunological defense mechanisms and thereby lead to the emergence of potentially antigenic neoplasms. Alternatively, regulatory mechanisms within the local microenvironment may exist that control the ability of resident epidermal LC to initiate and to elicit protective immunity against incipient cutaneous neoplasms. Indeed, APC may be critically involved in tumor immune surveillance, and the conditions within which the antigen is presented may determine the type and effectiveness of tumor immune responses in situ.[14] It has been shown that physical and functional alterations of cutaneous APC by UV irradiation as well as various cytokines can significantly modify the ability of epidermal APC to present TAA (discussed below). In this model, factors that are secreted by either the tumor cells themselves or by infiltrating host cells regulate tumor-antigen presentation and the effectiveness of the resulting immune response, providing a possible explanation for the capacity of antigenic tumors to grow progressively in situ. Thus, the fate of the immune response generated may be regulated on the level of antigen presentation.

NUMBER AND MORPHOLOGY OF DENDRITIC CELLS WITHIN TUMORS

In a traditional approach to evaluate the role of dendritic APC in tumor immunity, several investigators determined the number and morphology of dendritic cells within tumors or in their vicinity. Clinical studies revealed altered numbers and morphology of LC in the vicinity of epithelial malignancies and suggest a correlation between the number of tumor-infiltrating APC and clinical prognosis.[15,16] Interestingly, most, if not all agents with a known carcinogenic effect on cutaneous tissue also affect the morphology and function of epidermal LC.[17] In rats, tumor-infiltrating dendritic cells express high levels of MHC class I and class II, CD45, CD11a and intercellular adhesion molecule 1 (ICAM-1), but relatively low amounts of the costimulatory molecule B7-1. Moreover, a subpopulation of these cells also expresses the CD8 molecule.[18] A series of investigations performed by Halliday et al indicates that LC migrate into cutaneous neoplasms, possibly due to chemotactic effects of a tumor-derived cytokine.[19] However, no correlation between the LC number within cutaneous tumors and the type or degree of tumor immunity was found in this tumor system.[20] In contrast to human cancer patients,[11] tumor-bearing mice were not particularly susceptible to UVB-induced immunosuppression and did not display higher UV sensitivity of cutaneous LC in a murine melanoma model.[16,21] Thus, whereas morphological data favor a role for dendritic cells in tumor immunity, it is still uncertain whether cutaneous immunocompetence is relevant for tumor defense.

PRESENTATION OF TUMOR ANTIGENS BY DENDRITIC CELLS IN UNPRIMED AS WELL AS IN PRIMED SYSTEMS

Until recently, direct experimental evidence for the capacity of dendritic APC to present TAA was lacking. To address the role of epidermal APC in tumor immunity, initial studies showed that during the latent period of UV carcinogenesis, the number of identifiable epidermal LC decreased early in the course of chronic UV irradiation carcinogenesis, correlating with a decrease in antigen-presenting activity after sensitization through the UV-irradiated skin.[22] Later, it was demonstrated that splenic APC can bind tumor antigens in tumor-bearing mice,[23] and that dendritic cells indeed are capable of presenting tumor antigens for the generation of specific tumor immunity in a number of experimental systems (reviewed in refs. 10, 14). In this regard, Knight et al found that normal splenic dendritic cells induce immunity against a methylcholanthrene-induced tumor and that intravenous administration of dendritic cells also led to regression of established tumors.[24] Shimizu and co-workers later showed that splenic adherent cells were able to present tumor antigens for induction of tumor immunity in vivo. These authors found that APC remain functional in tumor-bearing mice despite the apparent downregulation of tumor immunity during late stages of tumor progression, but other investigators found both impaired and increased APC activity in tumor-bearing animals.[25-27]

Our own studies aimed to investigate directly whether epidermal APC have the capacity to present TAA and whether regulatory mechanisms exist that control induction or elicitation of T cell mediated tumor immune responses on the level of antigen presentation.[28-32] To study the conditions required for *sensitization* against TAA by epidermal APC, naive syngeneic mice were immunized with epidermal cells (enriched for MHC I-A+ LC) which had been pulsed with TAA derived from a murine spindle-cell tumor, S1509a. This immunization resulted in protective immunity against subsequent tumor challenge. However, preincubation of epidermal cells with granulocyte/macrophage colony-stimulating factor (GM-CSF) was required for induction of tumor immunity in this system. Crude fragments from tumor lysates were found to be a sufficient source of TAA. Additional experiments investigated the *elicitation* of tumor immunity with TAA-pulsed epidermal cells by measuring the specific delayed-type hypersensitivity (DTH) response after footpad injection of TAA-pulsed epidermal cells in mice that had previously been immunized against S1509a. We found that I-A⁺ epidermal APC are highly capable of eliciting S1509a-specific DTH responses, even without prior culture in GM-CSF. These findings have recently been confirmed by several investigators. For example, Flamand et al showed that dendritic cells induce a protective humoral immune response against a murine plasmocytoma,[33] and Cohen et al demonstrated that LC induce tumor-specific CTL responses in vitro, further supporting the concept that dendritic cells are capable of presenting tumor antigens to primed tumor-specific T cells.[34]

REGULATION OF TUMOR-ANTIGEN PRESENTATION

Since dendritic cells have been shown to be capable of presenting tumor antigens for the induction of effective tumor immunity in vivo and in vitro, the question arises as to why immunogenic tumors emerge at all, and how they manage to grow in the vicinity of fully competent dendritic cells. We thus hypothesized that cytokines may be crucially involved in the regulation of tumor-antigen presentation by epidermal APC, and that primary and secondary immune responses may be differentially modulated by these cytokines.

One of the cytokines that regulate tumor-antigen presentation by LC is GM-CSF, since preincubation of LC in GM-CSF was required for the ability of LC to initiate effective immunity against S1509a in unprimed mice. Thus, it is likely that LC in situ reside in an "immature" state, being relatively incapable of inducing primary immune responses, and that they acquire this activity only after stimulation with the appropriate cytokines.[9,28] Interleukin (IL) 1α, tumor necrosis factor α (TNF-α), interferon γ (IFN-γ) and transforming growth factor β (TGF-β) were unable to substitute for GM-CSF in our system and, surprisingly, most of these cytokines were found to inhibit tumor-antigen presentation by epidermal LC.[30-32] For example, coincubation of LC with GM-CSF plus TNF-α, IL-1α or IFN-γ inhibited or abrogated the GM-CSF-induced functional transition of "fresh" to "cultured" LC, and exposure of LC to IL-10 before culture in GM-CSF also in-hibited the acquisition of competence to induce tumor immunity. However, the mechanisms differ by which these cytokines alter LC tumor-antigen presentation. TNF-α appeared to reversibly affect the ability of LC to effectively encounter the tumor antigen, since incubation of LC after or instead of GM-CSF exposure led to loss of tumor-antigen presentation, whereas TNF-α had no effect when applied before incubation with GM-CSF or after exposure to tumor antigen.[30] In this system, IL-1α was found to downregulate tumor-antigen presentation by epidermal APC via stimulation of TNF-α release.[32] In contrast, IL-10 appears to act via downregulation of GM-CSF-induced LC maturation.[35] Recent data obtained by Larsen et al suggest that IFN-γ downregulates costimulatory molecules on LC, providing a possible mechanism of action of IFN-γ in our assays.[36] In our hands, TGF-β had no effects on tumor-antigen presentation by LC, despite its inhibitory functions on other APC.[32]

Interestingly, the ability of fresh or GM-CSF-cultured LC to elicit an anti-tumor DTH response in preimmunized mice was affected in a different way by these cytokines. Whereas TNF-α inhibited the ability of GM-CSF-cultured LC to induce tumor immunity in naive mice, it augmented their ability to elicit tumor-specific DTH responses in primed animals. In the primed system, IL-1α was found to inhibit elicitation of DTH by TAA-pulsed fresh or GM-CSF-exposed LC, while IFN-γ only inhibited antigen presentation by fresh LC.[31]

Further experiments aimed at examining the effects of UV radiation on tumor-antigen presentation by epidermal APC, since UV radiation is not only one of the most significant cutaneous carcinogens, but also has been shown to modulate cutaneous immune responses in other systems.[12] UV radiation dose-dependently inhibited the ability of epidermal APC both to induce as well as to elicit tumor immunity in the S1509a system. This effect was not due to acute cytotoxicity for LC and could not be inhibited to a significant extent by addition of anti-TNF-α antibody.[30]

Taken together, these data indicate that the local microenvironment in the vicinity of cutaneous tumors may be of significant importance for the ability of resident cutaneous APC to initiate and to elicit tumor immune responses. These experiments suggest that local cytokine concentrations during antigen encounter by APC as well as during their interaction with T cells either within the skin or after migration to the lymph node determine the type and effectiveness of T cell dependent tumor immune responses. Known effects of some cytokines on LC function are summarized in Table 9.2.

Other investigators addressed the question how cytokines regulate tumor immunity by local application of cytokines at tumor sites or by transfection of cytokine genes into tumor cells. Indeed,

Table 9.2. Cytokine effects on Langerhans cell function*

GM-CSF	– promotes LC viability and proliferation of LC precursors (in combination with TNF-α) – increases allostimulatory function of LC – increases LC presentation of protein antigen (in vitro/in vivo) and tumor antigen (in vivo) to unprimed but not to primed T cells – may downregulate LC antigen processing and presentation to primed T cell clones in mice (dependent upon mouse strains)
TNF-α	– promotes LC viability and proliferation of LC precursors (in combination with GM-CSF) – increases LC antigen presentation in primed but not in unprimed systems in vivo, may inhibit LC antigen presentation to primed T cells in vitro – reverses the GM-CSF-induced upregulation of antigen presentation in unprimed systems – inhibits/promotes LC migration (conflicting data)
IL-1α	– enhances LC migration, may be a chemotaxin for LC – may synergize with GM-CSF in upregulation of allostimulatory capacity – inhibits/enhances LC antigen presentation to unprimed or to primed T cell (depending on the experimental system)
IL-1β	– induces LC activation after exposure to antigen, may induce LC emigration out of the epidermis and morphologic changes of LC in situ after challenge with antigen
TGF-β	– inhibits allostimulatory function of cultured but not of fresh LC, does not inhibit LC presentation of tumor antigen to unprimed or primed T cells
IFN-γ	– inhibits LC antigen presentation to unprimed and possibly also to primed T cells – may mediate tolerance induction
IL-10	– inhibits LC function (in some experimental systems)

* Reproduced in part, with permission, from Grabbe S, Luger T. The skin as an immunological organ as well as a target for immune responses. In: Baart de la Faille H, Kater L, eds. Elsevier 1994.

cytokine-induced tumor rejection may also be mediated via APC. For example, it was hypothesized that the anti-tumor effects of IL-4 (after local injection or transfection of tumor cells) are mediated via recruitment of APC.[37] Indirect evidence suggests that in IL-2- or IFN-γ-transfected tumor cells, the generation of tumor immunity is also mediated by host APC.[38] Many other cytokines have also been found to induce tumor immunity after transfection of tumor-cell targets. However, in most cases it is not clear whether the transfection process as such induced tumor-cell fragility and facilitated the generation of concomitant tumor immunity, or whether induction of tumor immunity is a direct result of the transfected cytokine. Therefore, Dranoff et al transfected several tumor lines with a whole panel of cytokine genes and assessed their effects on both tumorigenicity and induction of tumor immunity.[39] Using a tumor system that does not induce concomitant immunity upon injection of mock-transfected or irradiated tumor cells, they found that only transfection with the IL-2 gene, but not with other cytokines, resulted in loss of tumorigenicity. Tumor immunity against the wild-type tumor could not be generated by transfection with any of the cytokines alone. However, specific immunity against the wild-type tumor was observed after cotransfection of tumor cells with IL-2 *and* GM-CSF, or after sublethal X-irradiation of tumor cells transfected with GM-CSF alone. These data indicate that for in vivo induction of tumor immunity, at least two conditions have to be fulfilled: (1) in vivo tumor-cell destruction (generated by IL-2 transfection or X-irradiation), and (2) stimulation of APC function in situ (induced by GM-CSF transfection). In another approach, GM-CSF was administered in vivo using biodegradable microspheres mixed with tumor cells, which again led to induction of tumor-specific immunity.[40] It is likely that this effect of GM-CSF is due to its stimulatory activity on the capacity of dendritic cells to present antigen.

Finally, the successful generation of tumor immunity by transfection of costimulatory molecules may also involve APC. By comparing tumor immunity induced by B7-transfected/MHC class I+ and B7-transfected/MHC class I− tumor cells, Huang et al demonstrated that bone marrow-derived APC, and not the transfected tumor cells themselves, are the relevant APC for MHC class I-restricted tumor immunity.[41]

ROLE OF T CELL SUBPOPULATIONS
IN TUMOR IMMUNITY

In most systems, tumor-specific immunity is mediated by T cells. The type of T cell response, however, varies between tumor systems and can involve CD4[+] and CD8[+] effector T cells as well as CD4[+] or CD8[+] T_S cells.[1] Consequently, the immune response generated by these T cells range from complete or partial tumor destruction to no effect or even enhancement of tumor growth. It has been shown that in most tumor models, optimal tumor-immune responses require the coordinate interaction of both CD4[+] and CD8[+] T cells.[1,42] In general, CD4[+] T cells transmit long-term immunological memory, recruit macrophages and other mononuclear cells via secretion of cytokines, and provide "help" for CD8[+] CTL effector cells, which together with macrophages are responsible for the actual tumor-cell killing.[43] The mechanisms of T cell memory are so far only partially understood and are reviewed elsewhere.[44] The "helper" function of CD4[+] T cells can largely be substituted by cytokines, especially by IL-2, since local administration of IL-2 to the tumor site (e.g., by transfection of tumor cells with the IL-2 gene) can bypass the requirement for CD4[+] T cell "help" to eradicate tumor cells.[45] However, in most systems IL-2 transfection does not reconstitute the generation of T cell memory and protective tumor immunity. Thus, CD8[+] effector T cells appear to require exogenous IL-2 for optimal CTL activity, which is provided by activated, tumor-specific CD4[+] cells in their vicinity.[43]

Besides effector T cells, many tumors also stimulate the clonal expansion of T cells that downregulate tumor immune responses, especially in advanced stages of malignant diseases. Until now, the phenotype and function of these T_S cells have not been characterized sufficiently. They may constitute a heterogeneous T cell population, since T_S cells have been attributed to the T helper type 2 (Th2) population, whereas in other systems they were found to be CD8[+] T cells.[1,46,47] Moreover, it is unclear whether there are distinct antigenic epitopes that lead to T_S induction, whether they are part of an idiotype/anti-idiotype network, or whether they recognize the same epitopes as effector T cells but secrete a different cytokine profile after activation, resulting in functional suppression of the tumor immune response.[47,48] Among the best-investigated models of T_S action is UV light-induced carcinogenesis. Studies performed by Kripke et al demonstrated that UV-induced skin tumors were generally poorly transplantable upon normal syngeneic hosts, but grew progressively if this host had been UV-irradiated prior to transplantation of the tumor (reviewed in refs. 10, 12). Transfer of splenic T cells from either tumor-bearing or from non-tumor-bearing, UV-irradiated mice led to a suppression of the ability of normal mice to reject UV radiation-induced tumors, indicating that the induction of T_S cells directed against epitopes on UV-induced tumors was responsible for the suppressed immune response by UV-irradiated hosts to these tumors. These T_S cells generally recognized UV-induced tumors as a group within a given strain of mice and did not affect non-UV-induced neoplasms (e.g., chemically induced tumors). Cloned UV-T_S cell lines have been established in vitro, which have some characteristics of Th2 cells.[49]

Taken together, these data show that T_S may be a heterogeneous population of T cells. In most cases, however, they are antigen-specific and MHC-restricted, indicating that their formation also requires antigen presentation. Thus, induction of tumor-specific tolerance may be due to altered or ineffective presentation of tumor antigens. Insufficient costimulatory signals may be responsible for the apparent lack of tumor immunity despite the presence of antigenic epitopes in some tumor systems.[50] Using epidermal LC as APC, it was demonstrated that in vitro UVB-irradiated epidermal APC lose their capacity to induce or elicit tumor-specific immune responses.[30] For protein antigens, it was shown that UVB irradiation converts LC from immunogenic to tolerogenic APC,[51] and recent observations from our laboratory suggest that a distinct subset of I-A$^+$ epidermal APC characterized by high buoyant density is capable of inducing tolerance to tumor antigens.[29] Interestingly, these cells lose their capacity to induce tolerance after culture in GM-CSF, indicating that tolerance can be induced by "immature" LC. These data further support the hypothesis that induction of immunity or tolerance depends upon the functional state of APC, which is greatly dependent upon an adequate cytokine microenvironment.

TUMOR IMMUNOTHERAPY BY MODULATION OF TUMOR-ANTIGEN PRESENTATION

The obvious goal of investigating the role of APC in tumor immunity is to evaluate their potential use as immunotherapeutic agents. Since dendritic cells can now be obtained in sizable numbers by culture of precursor cells from bone marrow or peripheral blood of mice as well as humans, this approach has become conceivable. Successful immunotherapy of established tumors has to achieve two major goals: (1) to induce tumor-specific immunity and (2) to overcome tumor-induced downregulation of immune responses. It has now been demonstrated in a number of tumor systems that tumor antigen-pulsed dendritic cells are potent inducers of specific tumor immunity, leading to effective protection against subsequent tumor challenge. Moreover, intratumoral injection of tumor antigen-pulsed dendritic cells resulted in regression of established tumors in this system.[52] However, it still needs to be determined whether this immunization strategy is able to bypass the numerous ways by which tumors induce downregulation of tumor immune reactions, such as by production of immunosuppressive cytokines, loss or mutation of antigenic epitopes and MHC molecules, shedding of soluble adhesion molecules, downregulation of costimulatory molecules on the surface of tumor-infiltrating APC, or induction of tumor-specific T_S cells. Indeed, tolerance induction may abrogate the possibility of subsequent immunization against tumors.[53] Another concern is the induction of autoimmune disease by immunization with tumor antigen-pulsed dendritic cells, since many immunogenic epitopes on tumors are not expressed exclusively by tumor cells but are also found in low amounts on the surface of normal cells. A recent study by Hu et al demonstrated, however, that the generation of autoimmune disease may not be a major obstacle in tumor immunotherapy.[53]

In summary, it has been formally shown that dendritic cells are able to present TAA for induction of protective tumor immunity in vivo. Moreover, an important role for dendritic APC in other models of tumor immunotherapy, such as by transfection of cytokines or costimulatory molecules, is now becoming apparent. However, further studies are necessary to obtain a more detailed understanding of tumor-antigen presentation in situ, and to evaluate the potential of dendritic cells as immunotherapeutic agents for tumor treatment.

REFERENCES

1. Mukherji B, Chakraborty NG, Sivanandham M. T-cell clones that react against autologous human tumors. Immunol Rev 1990; 116:33-62.
2. Becker JC, Schwinn A, Dummer R et al. Lesion-specific activation of cloned human tumor-infiltrating lymphocytes by autologous tu-

mor cells: induction of proliferation and cytokine production. J Invest Dermatol 1993; 101:15-21.

3. Pardoll DM. Tumour antigens. A new look for the 1990s. Nature 1994; 369:6479.

4. Slingluff CL, Hunt DF, Engelhard VH. Direct analysis of tumor-associated peptide antigens. Curr Opin Immunol 1994; 6:733-40.

5. Nagarkatti M, Clary SR, Nagarkatti PS. Characterization of tumor-infiltrating CD4+ T cells as Th1 cells based on lymphokine secretion and functional properties. J Immunol 1990; 144:4898-905.

6. Sprent J, Schaefer M. Capacity of purified Lyt-2+ T cells to mount primary proliferative and cytotoxic responses to Ia-tumour cells. Nature 1986; 322:541-4.

7. Kraig E, Kannapell C, Fischbach K et al. Two ultraviolet tumor-specific suppressor cell clones. J Immunol 1990; 145:2050-6.

8. Steinman RM. The dendritic cell system and its role in immunogenicity. Annu Rev Immunol 1991; 9:271-96.

9. Streilein JW, Grammer SF, Yoshikawa T et al. Functional dichotomy between Langerhans cells that present antigen to naive and to memory/effector T lymphocytes. Immunol Rev 1990; 117:159-83.

10. Grabbe S, Granstein RD. Mechanisms of ultraviolet radiation carcinogenesis. In: Granstein RD, ed. Mechanisms of Immune Regulation. Basel: Karger, 1994:291-313. (Adorini L, Ken-ichi A, Fitch FW et al, eds. Chemical Immunology; Vol 58).

11. Streilein JW. Immunogenetic factors in skin cancer. N Engl J Med 1992; 325:884-6.

12. Kripke ML. Immunologic mechanisms in UV-radiation carcinogenesis. Adv Cancer Res 1981; 34:69-106.

13. Ebbesen P, Kripke ML. Influences of age and anatomical site on ultraviolet carcinogenesis in BALB/c mice. J Natl Cancer Inst 1982; 68:691-4.

14. Grabbe S, Beissert S, Schwarz T et al. Dendritic cells as initiators of tumor immune responses: a possible strategy for tumor immunotherapy? Immunol Today 1995; 16:117-21.

15. Becker Y. Anticancer activity of dendritic cells. Symposium Proceedings of the Fourth International Conference of Anticancer Research. Crete. In Vivo 1993; 7:185-313.

16. Romerdahl CA, Okamoto H, Kripke ML. Immune surveillance against cutaneous malignancies in experimental animals. Immunol Ser 1989; 46:749-67.

17. Ruby JC, Halliday GM, Muller HK. Differential effects of benzo[a]pyrene and dimethylbenz[a]-anthracene on Langerhans cell distribution and contact sensitization in murine epidermis. J Invest Dermatol 1989; 92:150-5.

18. Chaux P, Hamann A, Martin F et al. Surface phenotype and functions of tumor-infiltrating dendritic cells: CD8 expression by a cell subpopulation. Eur J Immunol 1993; 23:2517-25.

19. Halliday GM, Lucas AD, Barnetson RSC. Control of Langerhans' cell density by a skin tumour-derived cytokine. Immunology 1992; 77:13-8.

20. Halliday GM, Reeve VE, Barnetson RSC. Langerhans cell migration into ultraviolet light-induced squamous skin tumors is unrelated to anti-tumor immunity. J Invest Dermatol 1991; 97:830-4.

21. Donawho CK, Kripke ML. Lack of correlation between UV-induced enhancement of melanoma development and local suppression of contact hypersensitivity. Exp Dermatol 1992; 1:20-6.

22. Alcalay J, Kripke ML. Antigen-presenting activity of draining lymph node cells from mice painted with a contact allergen during ultraviolet carcinogenesis. J Immunol 1991; 146:1717-21.

23. Shimizu J, Zou J-P, Ikegame K et al. Evidence for the functional binding in vivo of tumor rejection antigens to antigen-presenting cells in tumor-bearing hosts. J Immunol 1991; 146:1708-14.

24. Knight SC, Hunt R, Dore C et al. Influence of dendritic cells on tumor growth. Proc Natl Acad Sci USA 1985; 82:4495-7.

25. Shimizu J, Suda T, Yoshioka T et al. Induction of tumor-specific in vivo protective immunity by immunization with tumor antigen-pulsed antigen-presenting cells. J Immunol 1989; 142:1053-9.

26. Zou J, Shimizu J, Ikegame K et al. Tumor-bearing mice exhibit a progressive increase in tumor antigen-presenting cell function and a reciprocal decrease in tumor antigen-responsive CD4+ T cell activity. J Immunol 1992; 148:648-55.

27. Yamashita U. Dysfunction of Ia-positive antigen-presenting cells in tumor-bearing mice. Jpn J Cancer Res 1987; 78:261-9.

28. Grabbe S, Bruvers S, Gallo RL et al. Tumor antigen presentation by murine epidermal cells. J Immunol 1991; 146:3656-61.

29. Tan KC, Hosoi J, Grabbe S et al. Epidermal cell presentation of tumor-associated antigens for induction of tolerance. J Immunol 1994; 153:760-7.

30. Grabbe S, Bruvers S, Lindgren AM et al. Tumor antigen presentation by epidermal antigen-presenting cells in the mouse: modulation by granulocyte-macrophage colony stimulating factor, tumor necrosis factor α, and ultraviolet radiation. J Leukoc Biol 1992; 52:209-17.

31. Grabbe S, Bruvers S, Granstein RD. Effects of immunomodulatory cytokines on the presentation of tumor-associated antigens by epidermal Langerhans cells. J Invest Dermatol 1992; 99:66S-68S.

32. Grabbe S, Bruvers S, Granstein RD. Interleukin 1 alpha but not transforming growth factor beta inhibits tumor antigen presentation by epidermal antigen-presenting cells. J Invest Dermatol 1994; 102:67-73.

33. Flamand V, Sornasse T, Thielemans K et al. Murine dendritic cells pulsed in vitro with tumor antigen induce tumor resistance in vivo. Eur J Immunol 1994; 24:605-10.

34. Cohen PJ, Cohen PA, Rosenberg SA et al. Murine epidermal Langerhans cells and splenic dendritic cells present tumor-associated antigens to primed T cells. Eur J Immunol 1994; 24:315-9.

35. Beissert S, Hosoi J, Grabbe S et al. IL-10 inhibits tumor antigen presentation by epidermal antigen-presenting cells. J Immunol 1994; in press.
36. Larsen CP, Ritchie SC, Hendrix R et al. Regulation of immunostimulatory function and costimulatory molecule (B7-1 and B7-2) expression on murine dendritic cells. J Immunol 1994; 152:5208-19.
37. Bosco M, Giovarelli M, Forni M et al. Low doses of IL-4 injected perilymphatically in tumor-bearing mice inhibit the growth of poorly and apparently nonimmunogenic tumors and induce a tumor-specific immune memory. J Immunol 1990; 145:3136-43.
38. Bannerji R, Arroyo CD, Cordon-Cardo C et al. The role of IL-2 secreted from genetically modified tumor cells in the establishment of antitumor immunity. J Immunol 1994; 152:2324-32.
39. Dranoff G, Jaffee E, Lazenby A et al. Vaccination with irradiated tumor cells engineered to secrete murine granulocyte-macrophage colony-stimulating factor stimulates potent, specific, and long-lasting anti-tumor immunity. Proc Natl Acad Sci USA 1993; 90:3529-43.
40. Golumbek PT, Azhari R, Jaffee EM et al. Controlled release, biodegradable cytokine depots: a new approach in cancer vaccine design. Cancer Res 1993; 53:5841-4.
41. Huang AY, Golumbek P, Ahmadzadeh M et al. Role of bone marrow-derived cells in presenting MHC class I-restricted tumor antigens. Science 1994; 264:961-5.
42. Pardoll DM. New strategies for enhancing the immunogenicity of tumors. Curr Opin Immunol 1993; 5:719-25.
43. Topalain SL. MHC class II restricted tumor antigens and the role of CD4+ T cells in cancer immunotherapy. Curr Opin Immunol 1994; 6:741-5.
44. Sprent J. T and B memory cells. Cell 1994; 76:315-22.
45. Fearon ER, Pardoll DM, Itaya T et al. Interleukin-2 production by tumor cells bypasses T helper function in the generation of an antitumor response. Cell 1990; 60:397-403.
46. DiGiacomo A, North RJ. T cell suppressors of antitumor immunity. The production of Ly-1-,2+ suppressors of delayed sensitivity precedes the production of suppressors of protective immunity. J Exp Med 1986; 164:1179-92.
47. Bloom BR, Salgame P, Diamond B. Revisiting and revising suppressor T cells. Immunol Today 1992; 13:131-6.
48. Mutis T, Cornelissen YE, Datema G et al. Definition of a human suppressor T-cell epitope. Proc Natl Acad Sci USA 1994; 91:9456-60.
49. Roberts LK, Spellman CW, Warner NL. Establishment of a continuous T cell line capable of suppressing anti-tumor immune responses in vivo. J Immunol 1983; 131:514-9.
50. Chen L, Linsley PS, Hellstrom KE. Costimulation of T cells for tumor immunity. Immunol Today 1993; 14:483-6.

51. Simon JC, Tigelaar RE, Bergstresser PR et al. Ultraviolet B radiation converts Langerhans cells from immunogenic to tolerogenic antigen-presenting cells. J Immunol 1991; 146:485-91.
52. Zou JP, Shimizu J, Ikegame K et al. Tumor immunotherapy with the use of tumor antigen-pulsed antigen-presenting cells. Cancer Immunol Immunother 1992; 35:1-6.
53. Hu J, Kindsvogel W, Busby S et al. An evaluation of the potential to use tumor-associated antigens as targets for antitumor T cell therapy using transgenic mice expressing a retroviral tumor antigen in normal lymphoid tissues. J Exp Med 1993; 177:1681-90.

CHAPTER 10

LANGERHANS CELLS IN CUTANEOUS LEISHMANIASIS

Heidrun Moll, Stefanie Flohé, Christine Blank

INTRODUCTION

Human beings become infected with protozoan parasites of the genus *Leishmania* when an infected female sandfly is probing for blood. Thus, the skin is the parasite's site of entry into the mammalian host, where it exists in the obligatory intracellular form and resides in mononuclear phagocytes. The infection presents as a large variety of disease manifestations differing markedly in their severity. In cutaneous leishmaniasis, the infection may be asymptomatic or it may result in clinical symptoms ranging from self-healing localized ulcers to uncontrolled diffuse cutaneous lesions. The pathological changes that characterize the various forms of the disease reflect the balance between parasite multiplication, the immune response of the host and the resultant degenerative changes.[1]

The disease profiles seen in humans can be imitated by experimental infection of mice with *Leishmania major*, a causative agent of cutaneous leishmaniasis in man. Mice of genetically resistant inbred strains (e.g., C57BL/6) can contain the infection with cutaneous lesions healing spontaneously, whereas genetically susceptible mice (e.g., BALB/c) develop progressive disease with fatal impact. This model has granted valuable insights into the nature of the immunological mechanisms controlling the course of

The Immune Functions of Epidermal Langerhans Cells, edited by Heidrun Moll.

leishmaniasis, with important implications for other infectious diseases. It has been demonstrated that the outcome of infection with *Leishmania* depends on the efficiency of the host's immune response. The humoral immunity is not important for the in vivo control of leishmaniasis; on the other hand, evidence for the central role of cell-mediated immunity is compelling.[1,2] Both resistance and susceptibility to disease are mediated by CD4+ T cells, depending on their lymphokine production pattern. Secretion of interferon-γ (IFN-γ) by T-helper cells of type 1 (Th1) promotes protection, whereas the release of interleukin (IL) 4 and IL-10 by Th2-like CD4+ cells has been suggested to facilitate the spreading of the parasites. In addition, CD8+ cells may be involved in mediating recall responses and resistance to reinfection with *L. major*.[3] IFN-γ mediates the elimination of parasites via its stimulatory effect on macrophages, which can be counteracted by the deactivating cytokines IL-4, IL-10 and transforming growth factor β (TGF-β).[4]

Until recently, it was assumed that macrophages are the only type of cells with the ability to phagocytose *Leishmania* and to present parasite antigens to specific T cells. We have provided evidence that, in addition to macrophages, dendritic cells in the skin and in the lymph nodes draining the cutaneous lesion serve as host cells for the parasites and are critically involved in the immunoregulation of cutaneous leishmaniasis.[5] Therefore, murine infection with *L. major* is an excellent model to reveal the functions of epidermal Langerhans cells (LC) and other dendritic cells in infections with microorganisms that are handled by the endocytic pathway of the host cell (bacteria and parasites). In this chapter, we review our findings on the ability of LC and lymph node dendritic cells to interact with *L. major* and to stimulate a parasite-specific T-cell response, and we discuss the implications for the immunopathology and immune regulation of cutaneous leishmaniasis and related diseases.

INVOLVEMENT OF LANGERHANS CELLS
IN EARLY EVENTS OF CUTANEOUS LEISHMANIASIS

The first encounter of *Leishmania* parasites with the host's immune system takes place in the skin of the newly infected individual. At this location, there are two types of host cells that qualify as a sanctuary for the parasites—macrophages and epidermal LC—

because they express receptors for the complement component C3bi (CR3) which is used for attachment by the organisms. Whereas the role of macrophages as a scavenger of infectious agents is well-established, the ability of LC to phagocytose complex particles and contribute to resistance to infections has been revealed only recently.

Epidermal LC are considered to represent functionally immature dendritic cells that can stimulate primed T cells but are inefficient in presenting antigen to resting T cells. During short-term in vitro culture, they develop into cells resembling lymphoid dendritic cells and become very potent mediators of a primary T cell immune response. This differentiation presumably reflects the events in vivo, when antigen-bearing LC migrate from the skin to the regional lymph node. On the other hand, freshly isolated LC have the capacity to process protein antigens, a property that is lost during in vitro culture and differentiation into lymphoid dendritic cells.[6] Thus, phagocytic activity would be a useful skill to supply epidermal LC with antigen particles from pathogenic organisms for subsequent processing into peptides, loading of major histocompatibility complex (MHC) class II molecules and presentation to primed T cells, or, after differentiation into lymphoid dendritic cells, to naive T cells.

PHAGOCYTIC ACTIVITY OF LANGERHANS CELLS

When we investigated the phagocytic activity of LC, we found that freshly isolated LC (representing the intracutaneous state of differentiation), but not cultured LC (resembling lymphoid dendritic cells), can internalize *L. major* in vitro.[7] The parasites reside in phagosomes, and their uptake is mediated by the CR3. Both LC from mice that are genetically resistant to *L. major* infection and LC from susceptible mice are able to ingest the parasites, although their rate of infection in vitro differs slightly (C57BL/6: 8% ± 4%; BALB/c: 20.5% ± 5%). Parasite-containing LC are also present in vivo in the dermal infiltrate of lesional skin from *L. major*-infected mice[7] and from *L. mexicana*-infected patients (H. Moll and I. Becker, unpublished). These findings document that LC are able to phagocytose organisms of considerable size (2-5 μm) in vitro and in vivo. Uptake of microorganisms by LC has been demonstrated not only for *Leishmania* parasites but also for bacteria including *Staphylococcus aureus*,[8] mycobacteria[9] and *Borrelia burgdorferi* (M. Rittig, personal communication), and for yeasts.[8] We therefore suggest that LC should not be regarded as immature dendritic cells but rather as dendritic cells that are specialized for the uptake of particles and the processing of antigen, a task that matches well with their location in the skin which is the gateway for many pathogenic microorganisms.

ANTIGEN PRESENTATION BY LANGERHANS CELLS

Interestingly, the rate of infection and the parasite load of LC is much lower than that of macrophages. It is thus conceivable that phagocytosis of microorganisms by LC is not aimed at avid scavenging of the particles but at antigen processing and presentation, since occupancy of as few as 100 to 300 MHC class II molecules with antigenic peptides has been demonstrated to be sufficient for the stimulation of a T cell.[10] This concept was confirmed by our finding that LC are potent stimulators of *L. major*-specific T cell proliferation and lymphokine production in vitro.[11] In this respect, their efficiency was much greater than that of macrophages.

It has been suggested that the type of antigen-presenting cell (APC) may influence the development of Th-cell subsets producing discrete patterns of lymphokines.[12-14] Such an effect may be attributed to the release of particular cytokines and/or the relative levels of expression of costimulatory molecules by the APC. It was therefore of interest to determine whether presentation of *L. major* antigen by LC compared to macrophages elicits different lymphokine activities of the responding T cells. For analysis of this issue, we used a limiting dilution system that allows the quantitation of antigen-specific precursor T cells at the clonal level.[15] In these assays, LC stimulated *L. major*-specific T cells with the potential for production of IFN-γ and T cells with the potential for IL-4 release (Table 10.1), indicating that they are able to induce the development of both Th1 and Th2 cells. Macrophages, on the other hand, were more effective in the activation of *L. major*-reactive Th2-like cells with the capacity to secrete IL-4. In other systems, however, macrophages have been demonstrated to favor the development of Th1 cells.[13,14] These findings indicate that the nature of the accessory cell does not exclusively determine which Th-cell subset predominates and are in line with the suggestion that the presence of cytokines produced from other cells in the microenvironment is decisive for the type of developing Th cells.[16,17]

Table 10.1. Comparison of lymphokine production of L. major-reactive T cells after stimulation with either Langerhans cells or macrophages*

Type of APC	Reciprocal of frequency (95% confidence limits)	
	IFN-γ	IL-4
LC	7,936 (4,237-60,975)	6,241 (4,340-11,082)
Macrophages	>450,000	18,365 (11,417-46,657)

* Limiting numbers of lymph node cells from BALB/c mice immunized with *L. major* lysate were cultured with syngeneic LC or macrophages in the presence or absence of *L. major* antigen. Limiting dilution cultures were restimulated 7 days later, and, 24 hours thereafter, supernatants from individual cultures were collected and split for determination of lymphokine activities by ELISA. The number of cultures that were positive in the absence of antigen was subtracted from the fraction of cultures responding in the presence of antigen for each dose group. Estimates of the precursor frequencies were obtained by the minimum χ^2 method. The data represent mean values from two experiments. All *p* values >0.1.

ANTIGEN TRANSPORT AND INITIATION OF A PRIMARY T CELL RESPONSE

Dendritic cells do not directly promote the generation of a polarized Th1 or Th2 phenotype; however, there is substantial evidence that they are essential for priming and proliferation of naive T cells.[16,18,19] In the initial phase of cutaneous leishmaniasis, the delivery of a principal sensitizing signal seems to be the critical function of dendritic cells. This effect is directly connected with the migratory properties of LC. We observed that as early as 24-48 hours after intradermal infection with *L. major*, small numbers of dendritic cells carrying parasites appear in the draining lymph node.[20] Tracking experiments conducted in vivo using a stable fluorescence dye suggested that these cells are derived from epidermal LC that have taken up parasites in the skin. The ingestion takes place in the dermal compartment, since LC in the epidermis were never found to be infected. Thus, *Leishmania* infection results in an emigration of LC from the epidermis into the dermis, followed by phagocytosis of the organisms and transport to the draining lymph node. Most notably, the migratory dendritic cells have the capacity to activate resting T cells with specificity for *L. major* antigen.[20] Macrophages, on the other hand, are unable to carry parasite antigen from the skin to the lymph nodes and do not induce a primary T cell response.

Taken together, the distinctive function of LC in the early phase of cutaneous leishmaniasis in both susceptible and resistant mice appears to be the uptake of parasites in the dermis and their transport to the T cell areas of the local lymph node. During migration, LC develop into potent APC with the ability to stimulate selected, naive T cells for initiation of the immune response. Subsequently, activated T cells with specificity for *Leishmania* antigens emigrate from the lymph node via the blood to the infected skin, where parasitized macrophages and LC that remained in the lesion present antigen to the infiltrating T cells. The T cell effector activity is likely to be determined by the availability of cytokines that are produced locally by cells of the innate immune system. The presence of IL-12 and IFN-γ would induce the development of Th1 cells, whereas IL-4 directs the generation of Th2 cells.[21]

FUNCTIONS OF LYMPH NODE DENDRITIC CELLS IN MICE THAT HAVE RECOVERED FROM CUTANEOUS LEISHMANIASIS

After spontaneous recovery from cutaneous leishmaniasis, a long-lasting immunity protects mice of resistant strains from subsequent infections. Nevertheless, small numbers of intracellular parasites persist in the lymph nodes draining the site of the prior skin lesion.[3,22] It has been shown that the persistent organisms retain the karyotype, the general antigen-expression pattern and the degree of infectivity of the original inoculum. Persistence of *Leishmania* parasites has also been documented in humans, and situations of immunosuppression caused either by drug treatment or by infection with human immunodeficiency virus (HIV) may result in reactivation of the disease.[22]

PARASITE PERSISTENCE IN DENDRITIC CELLS

We examined whether dendritic cells, in addition to their critical role in the initiation of the immune response to *L. major*, also support the persistence of parasites in immune mice. Analysis of the phenotype of long-term host cells revealed that similar numbers of both macrophages and dendritic cells in the lymph nodes harbor viable *L. major* parasites which retain full virulence.[23] Strikingly, however, only lymph node dendritic cells but not macrophages are able to present endogenous antigen from persistent parasites to *L. major*-reactive T cells in vitro. Furthermore, they are extremely efficient because a small number of dendritic cells with a low parasite load is sufficient to trigger maximal T cell responses to *L. major*.

The impairment in the antigen-presenting capacity of long-term infected macrophages from immune mice may be attributed to a decreased expression of MHC class II molecules,[24] a defect in the intracellular loading of MHC class II molecules with antigenic peptides,[25] and/or to deficient expression of costimulatory molecules such as B7 and heat-stable antigen.[26] Conversely, the potent T cell stimulatory activity of dendritic cells carrying persistent parasites may be assigned to the constitutive expression of large amounts of MHC class II molecules[18] and the costimulatory molecule B7.[27] Another critical feature contributing to the efficient presentation of low amounts of persistent *L. major* antigen may be the ability of dendritic cells to cluster high numbers of T cells.[18]

Our data suggest that the lymph node dendritic cells harboring persistent parasites originate from the prior skin lesions of the recovered mice.[23] In fact, the observation that the local lymph nodes are the most consistent source of cryptic parasites[3,22] may be explained by the concept that those organs are the target of LC homing. Macrophages, which are not able to emigrate from the skin, may take up persistent organisms released by dendritic cells in the lymph node. Similarly, ingestion of parasites by resident lymph node dendritic cells may contribute to maintaining the frequency of infected cells. However, our previous finding that cultured LC, the in vitro equivalent of dendritic cells in lymphoid organs, have lost the ability to phagocytose *L. major*[7] argues against the latter possibility and indicates that all the lymph node dendritic cells containing *L. major* are derived from LC that have taken up the parasites *en route* in the dermal compartment.

PERSISTENT PARASITES—A ROLE IN THE MAINTENANCE OF T CELL MEMORY?

Persistence of virulent organisms has not only been reported for leishmaniasis but is also a well-known phenomenon for infections with mycobacteria[28] and with *Borrelia burgdorferi*.[29] An important question arising is that of the significance of pathogen persistence. In *immunocompetent* individuals, there may be an intricate balance between the low number of persistent microorganisms and the specific effector cells of the immune system that limit their replication. It is an intriguing idea that survival of a few pathogens may facilitate the maintenance of protective immunity. T cell memory may depend on perpetual restimulation mediated either by the continuous presence of antigen from the priming inoculum[30] or by cross-reactions with other pathogens.[31]

It should be emphasized that antigen persistence may not necessarily require the survival of virulent organisms but may also be based on residual antigenic peptides associated with MHC class II molecules. Dendritic cells are good candidates for such a long-term conservation of antigen because they shut down the biosynthesis of MHC class II products in the course of their differentiation from epidermal LC.[32-34] In vivo, this is likely to occur during migration from the skin to the draining lymph node. As a result, the MHC class II–peptide complexes of dendritic cells have a very long half-life, while those of macrophages turn over and decrease quickly.

In *immunocompromised* individuals, persistence of pathogens represents a serious health hazard. The reduced efficiency of the cell-mediated immunity results in the recurrence of latent infections. It remains to be shown whether relapsing leishmaniasis involves both the organisms persisting in dendritic cells and those residing in macrophages and whether this would have an effect on clinical manifestation, such as the tissue preferences of reactivated parasites.

MOLECULAR MECHANISMS
OF PARASITE HANDLING BY LANGERHANS CELLS

The findings described above suggest that dendritic cells have two major functions in cutaneous leishmaniasis: dendritic cells in the skin, i.e. LC, trigger the primary T cell response to *Leishmania* in the initial phase of infection, and lymph node dendritic cells are involved in the maintenance of immunity after recovery from infection. Macrophages, the major host cells for *Leishmania*, are not able to fulfil these tasks. The question arises whether these differences in the immunoregulatory functions of the two types of host cells correspond with differences in their interaction with the parasites. Whereas a large body of literature details the role of macrophages in resistance to infections and the mechanisms they use for destruction of invading microorganisms, there is no knowledge of the antimicrobial activities of LC or other dendritic cells. Therefore, it was of particular interest to study the pathways used by *Leishmania*-infected LC to restrict the replication of intracellular parasites and the factors involved in regulation of these activities. In addition, we examined the characteristics of *L. major*-infected LC that are related to their antigen-presentation function, i.e., the synthesis and turnover of MHC class II molecules and the associated invariant chain.

LEISHMANICIDAL ACTIVITIES OF LANGERHANS CELL

For *Leishmania*-infected macrophages, it has been demonstrated that intracellular killing of the parasites is mediated by nitric oxide (NO).[1,35] The synthesis of this reactive nitrogen intermediate from L-arginine is catalyzed by the inducible nitric oxide synthase (iNOS) that is triggered by cytokines, in particular IFN-γ, in synergy with lipopolysaccharide (LPS). Activated macrophages do not produce NO in the presence of N$^\omega$-monomethyl-L-arginine (L-NMMA), a substrate analogue for iNOS, and, as a result, parasite elimination is inhibited.

We studied the potential involvement of NO in the interaction between *L. major* and LC. In contrast to macrophages, the parasite load of infected LC was *not* increased in the presence of L-NMMA, the competitive inhibitor of iNOS, suggesting that the NO pathway does not contribute to the control of intracellular parasite replication by LC. This may be due to the lack of iNOS expression in LC and the use of other antimicrobial effector mechanisms. For analysis of this issue, epidermal cell suspensions were infected with *L. major* and/or treated with different cytokines in the presence or absence of LPS in vitro. Subsequently, pure LC were collected on the basis of morphological and phenotypical criteria, using single-cell picking, and were analyzed for expression of iNOS mRNA using the reverse transcriptase–polymerase chain reaction (RT-PCR). Activated macrophages were used as controls. In contrast to macrophages, expression of iNOS mRNA could not be induced in LC. While as few as 50 macrophages produced a significant signal, an almost hundredfold number of pure LC (4000 cells) did not display iNOS mRNA, either after stimulation with IFN-γ (Fig. 10.1) or various combinations of other cytokines in the presence or absence of LPS, or after infection with *L. major* (data not shown). On the other hand, high levels of iNOS mRNA

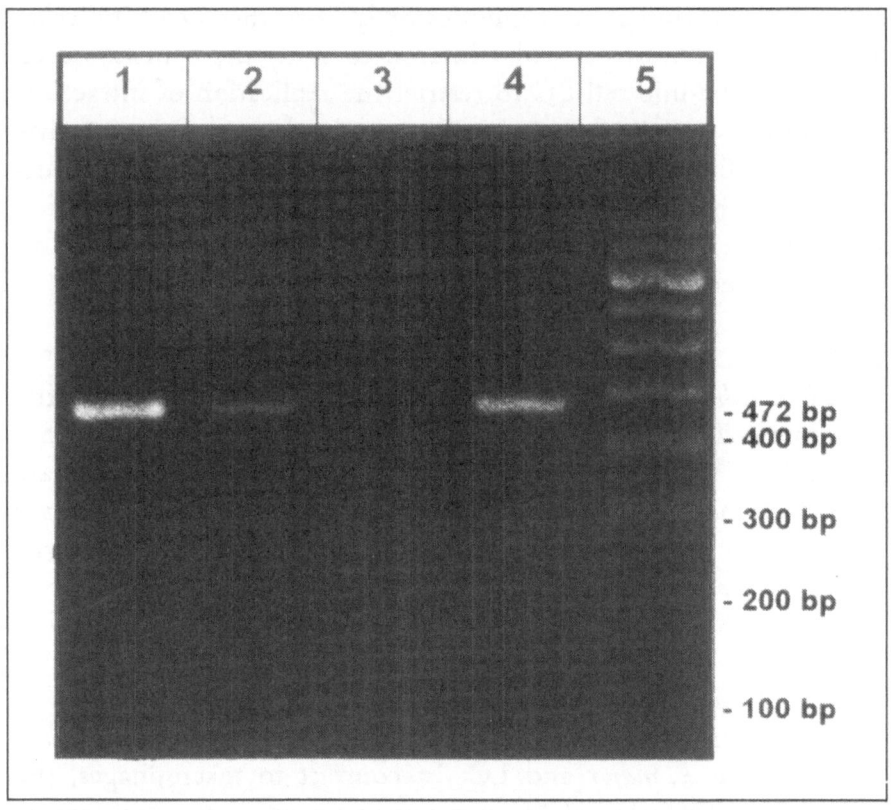

Fig. 10.1. Analysis of iNOS mRNA expression using RT-PCR. Epidermal cells were stimulated with IFN-γ, and macrophages were stimulated with IFN-γ and LPS in vitro. After 16 hours of incubation, cells were harvested for single-cell picking and preparation of mRNA. Lane 1: unselected epidermal cells (10[6] cells); lane 2: randomly picked, unselected epidermal cells (3000 cells); lane 3: LC (4000 cells); lane 4: J774 macrophages (50 cells); lane 5: DNA standard. Unstimulated cells gave no signal for iNOS mRNA and β-actin was detectable in all cells examined.

were detected in unselected epidermal cells (Fig. 10.1), a finding that is consistent with the previous observation that keratinocytes express this enzyme.[36]

Interestingly, however, previous findings demonstrated that LC are less permissive to infection with *L. major* than macrophages.[7] Thus, LC seem to restrict the growth of *L. major* by a mechanism that may not be mediated by iNOS and may therefore differ from the leishmanicidal pathway used by macrophages. In addition, the pathways appear to be regulated by different stimuli, because the restriction of intracellular parasite replication by LC, in contrast to macrophages, is not dependent on the presence of IFN-γ or tumor necrosis factor α (unpublished observations). It is possible that LC have the capacity to elicit oxidative burst activity, and the potential involvement of reactive oxygen intermediates in the antileishmanial response of LC is currently under investigation. Elucidation of this effector mechanism(s) will be of utmost importance for understanding the involvement of LC in infections with intracellular pathogens.

Finally, it should be emphasized that the observed failure of LC to express iNOS and, consequently, to produce reactive nitrogen intermediates, may be relevant not only for cutaneous leishmaniasis and the role of LC in resistance to infections, but also for other disease states. This notion is based on the fact that, in addition to its function as an antimicrobial effector molecule, NO is an important mediator of tumoricidal activity and has been implicated in processes of intercellular signalling.[37]

PATHWAYS OF *LEISHMANIA* ANTIGEN PRESENTATION BY LANGERHANS CELLS

The interaction between LC and *Leishmania* parasites or other intracellular pathogens is likely to be influenced by two factors. First, LC can display microbicidal effector activities that limit the growth of the invading organisms or kill them; second, LC efficiently process and present microbial antigen to specific T cells which, as a result of this stimulus, deliver soluble factors that modulate the antimicrobial activities of LC or other host cells.

In order to examine the characteristics of parasite antigen presentation by LC, we analyzed the antigen occupancy of MHC class II products as well as the biosynthesis and turnover of MHC class II molecules and the associated invariant chain in *L. major*-treated LC. For this purpose, LC that had been incubated in the presence or absence of *L. major* were pulse-labeled with ^{35}S-methionine, followed by sequential immunoprecipitation of MHC class II molecules and invariant chains and analysis by gel electrophoresis. Treatment with *L. major* resulted in the stable binding of peptides to MHC class II molecules corresponding with an enhanced formation of compact αβ dimers (C state)[38] that resist dissociation in sodium dodecyl sulfate (SDS). Furthermore, the half-life of MHC class II dimers loaded with parasite antigen was significantly longer in LC compared to macrophages. Most interestingly, however, incubation with *L. major* reduced the downregulation of the biosynthesis of MHC class II molecules that is observed during differentiation of LC in culture,[32-34] i.e., the expression of MHC class II products (α and β chains) was increased (Fig. 10.2, left part). We also observed the appearance of an additional band (25-28 kD) that we suppose to represent a degradation product of the associated invariant chain. On the other hand, incubation with *L. major* induced a decrease in the amounts of the free invariant chain forms p31 and p41 in LC (Fig. 10.2, right part). Both effects could not be observed after treatment of LC with a control

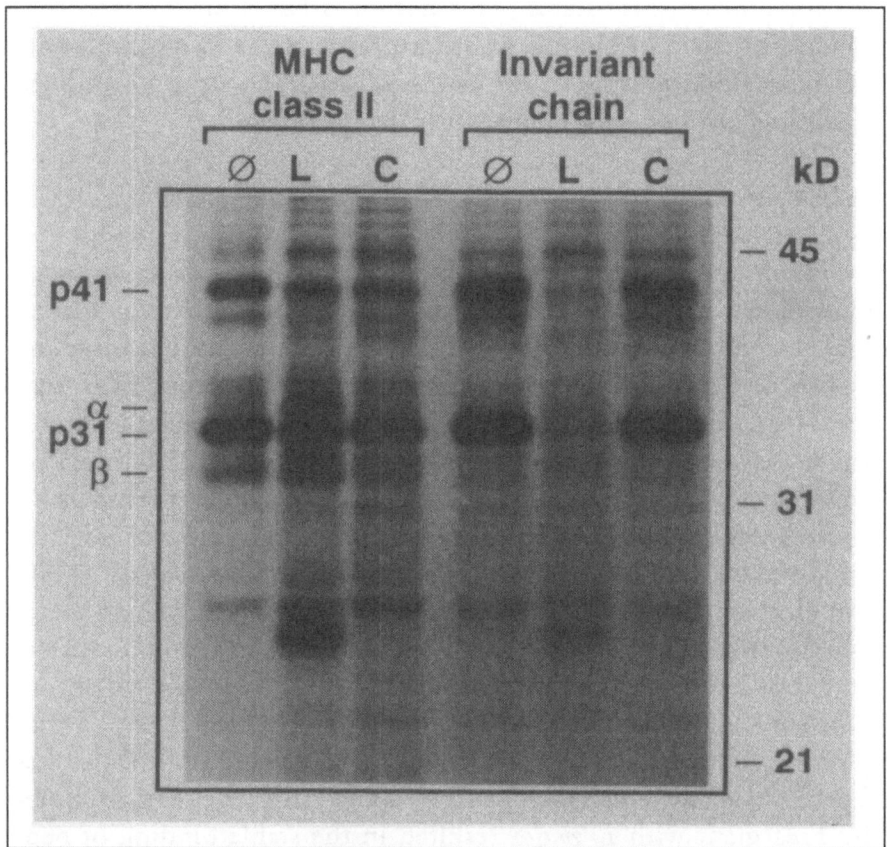

Fig. 10.2. Formation of MHC class II molecules and invariant chain forms in L. major-treated LC. Epidermal LC were cultured without antigen (Ø), or in the presence of L. major lysate (L) or myoglobin as a control antigen (C) for 8 hours, and, thereafter, were labeled with ³⁵S-methionine for 15 min. Subsequently, MHC class II molecules and associated invariant chains were immunoprecipitated with monoclonal antibody M5/114, against MHC class II (left part), and the remaining free invariant chain forms were immunoprecipitated with anti-invariant chain monoclonal antibody In-1 (right part). The samples were analyzed by sodium dodecyl sulfate-polyacrylamide gel electrophoresis (SDS-PAGE) followed by autoradiography.

antigen (myoglobin, Fig. 10.2) or after treatment of macrophages with either antigen (not shown). These findings indicate that *L. major* modifies the synthesis of MHC class II products and possibly also the formation of invariant chain forms in LC. As a result, the parasites may influence the antigen-presentation capacity of LC, thus modulating the host's immune response.

CONCLUDING REMARKS

In cutaneous leishmaniasis, both macrophages and LC/dendritic cells serve as host cells for the parasites and as APC for stimulation of a parasite-specific T cell response. When the various facets of these attributes are examined, however, considerable differences between macrophages and LC/dendritic cells become evident. Comparison of their spectrum of functional features shows that both types of cells fulfil specialized tasks (Table 10.2). Macrophages are the professional scavenger cells that carry a high load of parasites and, after appropriate activation, they are the effector cells for efficient intracellular killing of the organisms. On the other hand, the distinctive feature of LC in the initial phase of infection is the transport of ingested parasites from the skin to the draining lymph node, where they present *Leishmania* antigen to naive T cells for initiation of the specific immune response. At later stages, after cure of cutaneous lesions in mice that have become immune to reinfection, persisting parasites are sequestered in both macrophages and dendritic cells. However, only dendritic cells have the ability to present endogenous parasite antigen to T cells and may thus allow the sustained stimulation of parasite-specific memory T cells protecting the mice from reinfection.

Elucidation of the precise mechanisms underlying the processing of *Leishmania* antigen, the intracellular killing or growth restriction of the parasites, and the maintenance of protective T cells by LC/dendritic cells will be of considerable interest for the design of immunotherapeutic agents or vaccination strategies against infectious diseases. The unique accessory and migratory properties of LC/dendritic cells make them good candidates for use as antigen vehicles that provoke a specific T cell immune response. The recent advancements in generating dendritic cell lines and deriving sizeable numbers of human LC from peripheral blood offer greatly improved conditions for the development of new approaches.

Table 10.2. Functional features of Langerhans cells
compared to macrophages in experimental infection with L. major

	LC	Macrophages
Phagocytosis:		
Involvement of CR3	yes	yes
Involvement of MFR	no	yes
Rate of infection	+	+++
Parasite load	+	+++
Antigen presentation:		
Efficiency	+++	+/++
Induction of primary T cell response	yes	no
Induction of secondary T cell response	yes	yes
Increased expression of MHC class II	yes	no
Antigen transport (skin to lymph node):	yes	no
Parasite persistence:		
Long-term host cells	yes (DC)	yes
Presentation of endogenous antigen to		
specific T cells	yes (DC)	no
Effector mechanisms:		
RNI production	no	yes
ROI production	?	yes

CR3: complement component C3bi; DC: dendritic cells; MFR: mannose-fucose receptor;
RNI: reactive nitrogen intermediates. ROI: reactive oxygen intermediates.

ACKNOWLEDGMENTS

This work was supported by the Deutsche Forschungsgemein-schaft, Germany (DFG grant SFB263/A2), and by the Bundes-ministerium für Forschung und Technologie, Germany (BMFT grant KI 8906/0).

REFERENCES

1. Liew FY, O'Donnell CA. Immunology of leishmaniasis. Adv Parasitol 1993; 32:161-259.
2. Reed SG, Scott P. T-cell cytokine responses in leishmaniasis. Curr Opin Immunol 1993; 5:524-31.
3. Müller I. Role of T cell subsets during the recall of immunologic memory to *Leishmania major*. Eur J Immunol 1992; 22:3063-9.
4. Bogdan C, Gessner A, Röllinghoff M. Cytokines in leishmaniasis: a complex network of stimulatory and inhibitory interactions. Immunobiol 1993; 189:356-96.
5. Moll H. Epidermal Langerhans cells are critical for immunoregulation

of cutaneous leishmaniasis. Immunol Today 1993; 14:383-7.

6. Romani N, Schuler G. The immunologic properties of epidermal Langerhans cells as a part of the dendritic cell system. Springer Semin Immunopathol 1992; 13:265-79.

7. Blank C, Fuchs H, Rappersberger K et al. Parasitism of epidermal Langerhans cells in experimental cutaneous leishmaniasis with *L. major*. J Infect Dis 1993; 167:418-25.

8. Reis e Sousa C, Stahl PD, Austyn JM. Phagocytosis of antigens by Langerhans cells in vitro. J Exp Med 1993; 178:509-19.

9. Poulter LW, Collings LA, Tung KS et al. Parasitism of antigen-presenting cells in hyperbacillary leprosy. Clin Exp Med 1984; 55:611-7.

10. Harding CV. Pathways of antigen processing. Curr Opin Immunol 1991; 3:3-9.

11. Will A, Blank C, Röllinghoff M et al. Murine epidermal Langerhans cells are potent stimulators of an antigen-specific T cell response to *Leishmania major*, the cause of cutaneous leishmaniasis. Eur J Immunol 1992; 22:1341-7.

12. Chang TL, Shea CM, Urioste S et al. Heterogeneity of helper/inducer T lymphocytes. III. Responses of IL-2- and IL-4-producing (Th1 and Th2) clones to antigens presented by different accessory cells. J Immunol 1990; 145:2803-8.

13. Gajewski TF, Pinnas M, Wong T et al. Murine Th1 and Th2 clones proliferate optimally in reponse to distinct antigen-presenting cell populations. J Immunol 1991; 146:1750-8.

14. Schmitz J, Assenmacher M, Radbruch A. Regulation of T helper cell cytokine expression: functional dichotomy of antigen-presenting cells. Eur J Immunol 1993; 23:191-9.

15. Moll H, Röllinghoff M. Resistance to murine cutaneous leishmaniasis is mediated by T_H1 cells, but disease-promoting CD4+ cells are different from T_H2 cells. Eur J Immunol 1990; 20:2067-74.

16. Macatonia SE, Hsieh CS, Murphy KM et al. Dendritic cells and macrophages are required for Th1 development of CD4+ T cells from αβ TCR transgenic mice: IL-12 substitution for macrophages to stimulate IFN-γ production is IFN-γ-dependent. Int Immunol 1993; 5:1119-28.

17. Seder RA, Paul WE, Davis MM et al. The presence of interleukin 4 during in vitro priming determines the lymphokine-producing potential of CD4+ T cells from T cell receptor transgenic mice. J Exp Med 1992; 176:1091-8.

18. Steinman RM. The dendritic cell system and its role in immunogenicity. Annu Rev Immunol 1991; 9:271-96.

19. Croft M, Duncan DD, Swain SL. Response of naive antigen-specific CD4+ T cells in vitro: characteristics and antigen-presenting cell requirements. J Exp Med 1992; 176:1431-7.

20. Moll H, Fuchs H, Blank C et al. Langerhans cells transport *Leishmania major* from the infected skin to the draining lymph node for presentation to antigen-specific T cells. Eur J Immunol 1993; 23:1595-1601.

21. O'Garra A, Murphy K. Role of cytokines in determining T-lymphocyte function. Curr Opin Immunol 1994; 6:458-66.

22. Aebischer T. Recurrent cutaneous leishmaniasis: a role for persistent parasites? Parasitol Today 1994; 10:25-8.

23. Moll H, Flohé S, Röllinghoff M. Dendritic cells in *Leishmania major*-immune mice harbor persistent parasites and mediate an antigen-specific T-cell immune response. Eur J Immunol 1995; 25:693-9.

24. Reiner NE, Ng W, McMaster WR. Parasite-accessory cell interactions in murine leishmaniasis. II. *Leishmania donovani* suppresses macrophage expression of class I and class II major histocompatibility gene products. J Immunol 1987; 138:1926-32.

25. Fruth U, Solioz N, Louis JA. *Leishmania major* interferes with antigen presentation by infected macrophages. J Immunol 1993; 150:1857-64.

26. Kaye PM, Rogers NJ, Curry AJ et al. Deficient expression of co-stimulatory molecules on *Leishmania*-infected macrophages. Eur J Immunol 1994; 24:2850-4.

27. Larsen CP, Ritchie SC, Pearson TC et al. Functional expression of the costimulatory molecule, B7/BB1, on murine dendritic cell populations. J Exp Med 1992; 176:1215-20.

28. Britton WJ, Roche PW, Winter N. Mechanisms of persistence of mycobacteria. Trends Microbiol 1994; 2:284-8.

29. Preac-Mursic V, Weber K, Pfister HW et al. Survival of *Borrelia burgdorferi* in antibiotically treated patients with Lyme borreliosis. Infection 1989; 17:355-9.

30. Gray D, Matzinger P. T cell memory is short-lived in the absence of antigen. J Exp Med 1991; 174:969-74.

31. Selin LK, Nahill SR, Welsh RM. Cross-reactivities in memory cytotoxic T lymphocyte recognition of heterologous viruses. J Exp Med 1994; 179:1933-43.

32. Puré E, Inaba K, Crowley MT et al. Antigen processing by epidermal Langerhans cells correlates with the level of biosynthesis of major histocompatibility complex class II molecules and expression of invariant chain. J Exp Med 1990; 172:1459-69.

33. Becker D, Reske-Kunz AB, Knop J et al. Biochemical properties of MHC class II molecules endogenously synthesized and expressed by mouse Langerhans cells. Eur J Immunol 1991; 21:1213-20.

34. Kämpgen E, Koch N, Koch F et al. Class II major histocompatibility complex molecules of murine dendritic cells: synthesis, sialylation of invariant chain, and antigen processing capacity are down-regulated upon culture. Proc Natl Acad Sci USA 1991; 88:3014-8.

35. Green SJ, Crawford RM, Hockmeyer JT et al. *Leishmania major* amastigotes initiate the L-arginine-dependent killing mechanism in IFN-γ-stimulated macrophages by induction of tumor necrosis factor-α. J Immunol 1990; 145:4290-7.

36. Heck DE, Laskin DL, Gardner CR et al. Epidermal growth factor suppresses nitric oxide and hydrogen peroxide production by keratinocytes. J Biol Chem 1992; 267:21277-80.
37. Nathan C. Nitric oxide as a secretory product of mammalian cells. FASEB J 1992; 6:3051-64.
38. Germain RN, Hendrix LR. MHC class II structure, occupancy and surface expression determined by post-endoplasmic reticulum antigen binding. Nature 1991; 353:134-9.

QUESTIONNAIRE

Receive a FREE BOOK of your choice

Please help us out—Just answer the questions below, then select the book of your choice from the list on the back and return this card.

R.G. Landes Company publishes five book series: *Medical Intelligence Unit, Molecular Biology Intelligence Unit, Neuroscience Intelligence Unit, Tissue Engineering Intelligence Unit* and *Biotechnology Intelligence Unit*. We also publish comprehensive, shorter than book-length reports on well-circumscribed topics in molecular biology and medicine. The authors of our books and reports are acknowledged leaders in their fields and the topics are unique. Almost without exception, there are no other comprehensive publications on these topics.

Our goal is to publish material in important and rapidly changing areas of bioscience for sophisticated scientists. To achieve this goal, we have accelerated our publishing program to conform to the fast pace in which information grows in bioscience. Most of our books and reports are published within 90 to 120 days of receipt of the manuscript.

Please circle your response to the questions below.

1. We would like to sell our *books* to scientists and students at a deep discount. But we can only do this as part of a prepaid subscription program. The retail price range for our books is $59-$99. Would you pay $196 to select four *books* per year from any of our Intelligence Units–$49 per book–as part of a prepaid program?

                                                Yes   **No**

2. We would like to sell our *reports* to scientists and students at a deep discount. But we can only do this as part of a prepaid subscription program. The retail price range for our reports is $39-$59. Would you pay $145 to select five *reports* per year–$29 per report–as part of a prepaid program?

                                                Yes   **No**

3. Would you pay $39–the retail price range of our books is $59-$99–to receive any single book in our Intelligence Units if it is spiral bound, but in every other way identical to the more expensive hardcover version?

                                                Yes   **No**

To receive your free book, please fill out the shipping information below, select your free book choice from the list on the back of this survey and mail this card to:

    R.G. Landes Company, 909 S. Pine Street, Georgetown, Texas 78626 U.S.A.

Your Name _____

Address _____

City _____ State/Province: _____

Country: _____ Postal Code: _____

My computer type is Macintosh_____ ; IBM-compatible _____ ; Other _____

Do you own ____ or plan to purchase ___ a CD-ROM drive?

Available Free Titles

Please check three titles in order of preference.
Your request will be filled based on availability. Thank you.

☐ Water Channels
Alan Verkman,
University of California-San Francisco

☐ The Na,K-ATPase:
Structure-Function Relationship
J.-D. Horisberger, University of Lausanne

☐ Intrathymic Development of T Cells
J. Nikolic-Zugic,
Memorial Sloan-Kettering Cancer Center

☐ Cyclic GMP
Thomas Lincoln, University of Alabama

☐ Primordial VRM System and the Evolution
of Vertebrate Immunity
John Stewart, Institut Pasteur-Paris

☐ Thyroid Hormone Regulation
of Gene Expression
Graham R. Williams, University of Birmingham

☐ Mechanisms of Immunological Self Tolerance
Guido Kroemer, CNRS Génétique Moléculaire et
Biologie du Développement-Villejuif

☐ The Costimulatory Pathway
for T Cell Responses
Yang Liu, New York University

☐ Molecular Genetics of Drosophila Oogenesis
Paul F. Lasko, McGill University

☐ Mechanism of Steroid Hormone Regulation
of Gene Transcription
M.-J. Tsai & Bert W. O'Malley, Baylor University

☐ Liver Gene Expression
François Tronche & Moshe Yaniv,
Institut Pasteur-Paris

☐ RNA Polymerase III Transcription
R.J. White, University of Cambridge

☐ src Family of Tyrosine Kinases in Leukocytes
Tomas Mustelin, La Jolla Institute

☐ MHC Antigens and NK Cells
Rafael Solana & Jose Peña,
University of Córdoba

☐ Kinetic Modeling of Gene Expression
James L. Hargrove, University of Georgia

☐ PCR and the Analysis of the T Cell Receptor
Repertoire
Jorge Oksenberg, Michael Panzara & Lawrence
Steinman, Stanford University

☐ Myointimal Hyperplasia
Philip Dobrin, Loyola University

☐ Transgenic Mice as an In Vivo Model
of Self-Reactivity
David Ferrick & Lisa DiMolfetto-Landon,
University of California-Davis and Pamela Ohashi,
Ontario Cancer Institute

☐ Cytogenetics of Bone and Soft Tissue Tumors
Avery A. Sandberg, Genetrix & Julia A. Bridge ,
University of Nebraska

☐ The Th1-Th2 Paradigm and Transplantation
Robin Lowry, Emory University

☐ Phagocyte Production and Function Following
Thermal Injury
Verlyn Peterson & Daniel R. Ambruso,
University of Colorado

☐ Human T Lymphocyte Activation Deficiencies
José Regueiro, Carlos Rodríguez-Gallego
and Antonio Arnaiz-Villena,
Hospital 12 de Octubre-Madrid

☐ Monoclonal Antibody in Detection and
Treatment of Colon Cancer
Edward W. Martin, Jr., Ohio State University

☐ Enteric Physiology of the Transplanted Intestine
Michael Sarr & Nadey S. Hakim, Mayo Clinic

☐ Artificial Chordae in Mitral Valve Surgery
Claudio Zussa, S. Maria dei Battuti Hospital-Treviso

☐ Injury and Tumor Implantation
Satya Murthy & Edward Scanlon,
Northwestern University

☐ Support of the Acutely Failing Liver
A.A. Demetriou, Cedars-Sinai

☐ Reactive Metabolites of Oxygen and Nitrogen
in Biology and Medicine
Matthew Grisham, Louisiana State-Shreveport

☐ Biology of Lung Cancer
Adi Gazdar & Paul Carbone,
Southwestern Medical Center

☐ Quantitative Measurement
of Venous Incompetence
Paul S. van Bemmelen, Southern Illinois University
and John J. Bergan, Scripps Memorial Hospital

☐ Adhesion Molecules in Organ Transplants
Gustav Steinhoff, University of Kiel

☐ Purging in Bone Marrow Transplantation
Subhash C. Gulati,
Memorial Sloan-Kettering Cancer Center

☐ Trauma 2000: Strategies for the New Millennium
David J. Dries & Richard L. Gamelli,
Loyola University

CHAPTER 11

LANGERHANS CELLS AND HIV INFECTION

Colette Dezutter-Dambuyant, Anne-Sophie Charbonnier,
Marie-Madeleine Fiers, Pascale Delorme,
Nathalie Dusserre, Catherine Tsagarakis,
Claude Desgranges, François Mallet, Daniel Schmitt

INTRODUCTION

The skin and mucosa are the first line of defense of the organism against external agents, not only as a physical barrier between the body and the environment but also as the site of initiation of immune reactions. The immunocompetent cells which act as antigen-presenting cells are Langerhans cells (LC). Originating in the bone marrow, LC migrate to the peripheral epithelia (skin, mucous membranes) where they play a primordial role in the induction of an immune response and are especially active in stimulating naive T lymphocytes in the primary response through a specific cooperation with CD4-positive lymphocytes after migration to proximal lymph nodes. Apart from many plasma membrane determinants, LC also express CD4 molecules which make them a susceptible target and reservoir for human immunodeficiency virus type 1 (HIV-1). Once infected, these cells, due to their localization in areas at risk (skin, mucous membranes), to their ability to migrate from the epidermal compartment to lymph nodes and to their ability to support viral replication without major cytopathic effects, could play a role as a vector in the dissemination of virus

The Immune Functions of Epidermal Langerhans Cells, edited by Heidrun Moll.
© 1995 R.G. Landes Company.

from the site of inoculation to the lymph nodes, and may thereby contribute to the infection of T lymphocytes. The in vivo consequences resulting from LC infection in the pathobiology of HIV will be discussed.

EPIDERMAL LANGERHANS CELLS
ARE HIV-INFECTED IN VIVO

Acquired immunodeficiency syndrome (AIDS) is a disease characterized by profound immunosuppression with diverse clinical syndromes caused by a retrovirus called human immunodeficiency virus (HIV). HIV is a member of the lentivirus family of animal retroviruses which include the visna virus of sheep, and the bovine, feline and simian immunodeficiency viruses. Between 1984 and 1987, several authors suggested that LC could be implicated in the pathobiology of HIV, as the absolute number of epidermal LC in the epidermis of patients with AIDS or AIDS-related complex (ARC)[1] and in oral mucous lesions associated with AIDS[2] was significantly reduced. The disappearance appeared to be correlated with a decrease in the numbers of circulating CD4+ cells[3] as well as the clinical stage of the illness.[1]

Since 1987, different groups[4-6] have published electron microscope studies on skin from HIV-positive patients, in whom HIV particles have been observed in close proximity to LC. Furthermore, buds of retroviral particles from LC membrane have been observed in the same sample.[5] In some seropositive patients (7 out of 40 patients studied), monoclonal antibodies directed against HIV-1 gag proteins p17 and p24 were able to label epidermal cells. At the same time, the expression of CD4 antigens by LC has been investigated and in certain clinical conditions (ARC), an upregulated expression has been reported.[6] Epidermal sheets obtained from seropositive patients can transmit the virus after coculture with peripheral blood lymphocytes.[7] Thus, several indirect pieces of evidence have been acquired concerning the infection of LC by HIV. Certain studies were unable to demonstrate the presence of virus or viral proteins at the cutaneous level.[8] Such discrepancies are mainly due to the existence of individual variability as well as different anatomical localizations and immunohistochemistry sensitivity. In a transgenic mouse model, the HIV-1 long-terminal repeat (LTR) promoter controlling a reporter gene is preferentially expressed in some epithelial dendritic cells (i.e.,

LC) and can be activated by ultraviolet light[9,10] or skin-sensitizing chemicals.[11] Using techniques offering high sensitivity, such as in situ hybridization and polymerase chain reaction (PCR), some authors demonstrated the presence of HIV-1 proviral DNA sequences in the epidermis of seropositive patients and suggested the possibility of in vivo infection of LC,[12-15] whereas other investigators found no evidence for virus infection.[16]

The conflicting results could be accounted for by the methods used for the dermo-epidermal dissociation (chemical/enzymatic procedures[12,15] or suction blister[13]) or for the purification of LC suspensions.[14] As the dermal compartment in clinical specimens may contain a great variety of cell types from peripheral blood which are potentially HIV-infected, we selected a technique for a clean detachment of the epidermal compartment to avoid any contamination of either the dermal or epidermal compartments. The epidermal compartment was then analyzed for the presence of HIV DNA. A nondenaturating DNA was obtained from epidermal sheets after thermochemical treatment of biopsies (0.5 M ethylenediaminetetraacetic acid (EDTA), pH 7.5 at 60°C for 90 seconds). Optimization of amplification of viral genome was performed with three primer pairs derived from *gag*, *env*, and *pol* sequences. PCR products were analyzed by Southern blot. Viral genome was found in 5 out of 11 HIV-seropositive patients. These results corroborate previous studies where, using PCR, HIV-genome material was detected successively within the epidermal and dermal samples evaluated separately,[12] in epidermal cells collected by suction blister procedure,[13] and in highly purified LC by immunomagnetic separation.[14] Recently, epidermal LC from seropositive patients were shown to actively transcribe HIV-1 proviral DNA[17] and to be able to infect peripheral blood mononuclear cells from healthy donors in vitro,[18] although the frequency of infected LC is very low (107 to 3,645 HIV-1 DNA copies/10^5 LC).[17] Taken together, these results clearly demonstrated the presence of viral genome in the epidermal cells (highly suspected to be LC) which have the capacity to effectively transmit the virus to infectable cells.[19]

IN VITRO INFECTION
OF EPIDERMAL LANGERHANS CELLS

Between 1989 and 1991, we were able to demonstrate the capacity of normal LC to bind and to internalize HIV-1 gp120 or gp160 recombinant proteins in vitro.[20] This internalization occurs by receptor-mediated endocytosis (Fig. 11.1) and by Birbeck granules progressively induced from the plasma membrane (Fig. 11.2).[21] In suspensions of epidermal LC obtained by trypsinization of dermo-epidermal sheets, the binding of viral glycoproteins occurs via membrane receptor(s) that are different from CD4 molecules, since these latter molecules are cleaved and released during the preparation of epidermal LC.[20] Furthermore, receptors resistant to trypsin which are involved in the binding of viral glycoproteins are upregulated within 24 hours following isolation, whilst the cleaved CD4 are internalized from LC membranes and are not resynthesized. In vitro, gp120 internalization may be the result of complex interactions occurring between viral envelope proteins and cellular factors in addition to the gp120/CD4 interactions.[21]

In 1988, Braathen et al tested in vitro infection by incubation of LC-enriched epidermal cell suspensions with HIV-containing supernatant from an infected cell line. After four to five days of culture, some epidermal cells expressed p24 or gp120 viral proteins as demonstrated by immunocytochemical staining.[22] In vitro, no electron microscope studies have demonstrated LC permissiveness to replication of HIV. We developed an infection procedure to investigate the infection mechanism and to provide evidence that LC present in partially purified populations of epidermal cells can be infected in culture. We followed the morphological sequence of events when isolated LC were exposed for various time periods to HIV-1-carrying U937 monocytes (HIV-IIIB isolate). We demonstrated that LC were also capable of binding and internalizing viral particles by receptor-mediated endocytosis (Fig. 11.3).[15,23] Such an observation was made within the first three hours of the coculture. The route of entry of virus was shown to be identical to that of envelope proteins; nevertheless, the mechanism of fusion cannot be excluded since this latter is extremely rapid and consequently difficult to observe by electron microscopy. By prolonging the time of coculture of LC with the infected promonocytic cells, the LC show signs of permissiveness to replication. After four days of coculture, HIV-1 was clearly seen budding and being released from epidermal LC (Fig. 11.4).[24]

Recently, we experimentally infected epidermal LC with HIV-1 provided by a cell-free infection system.[25] Viral particles were made cell-free by low-speed centrifugation followed by 0.45 µm

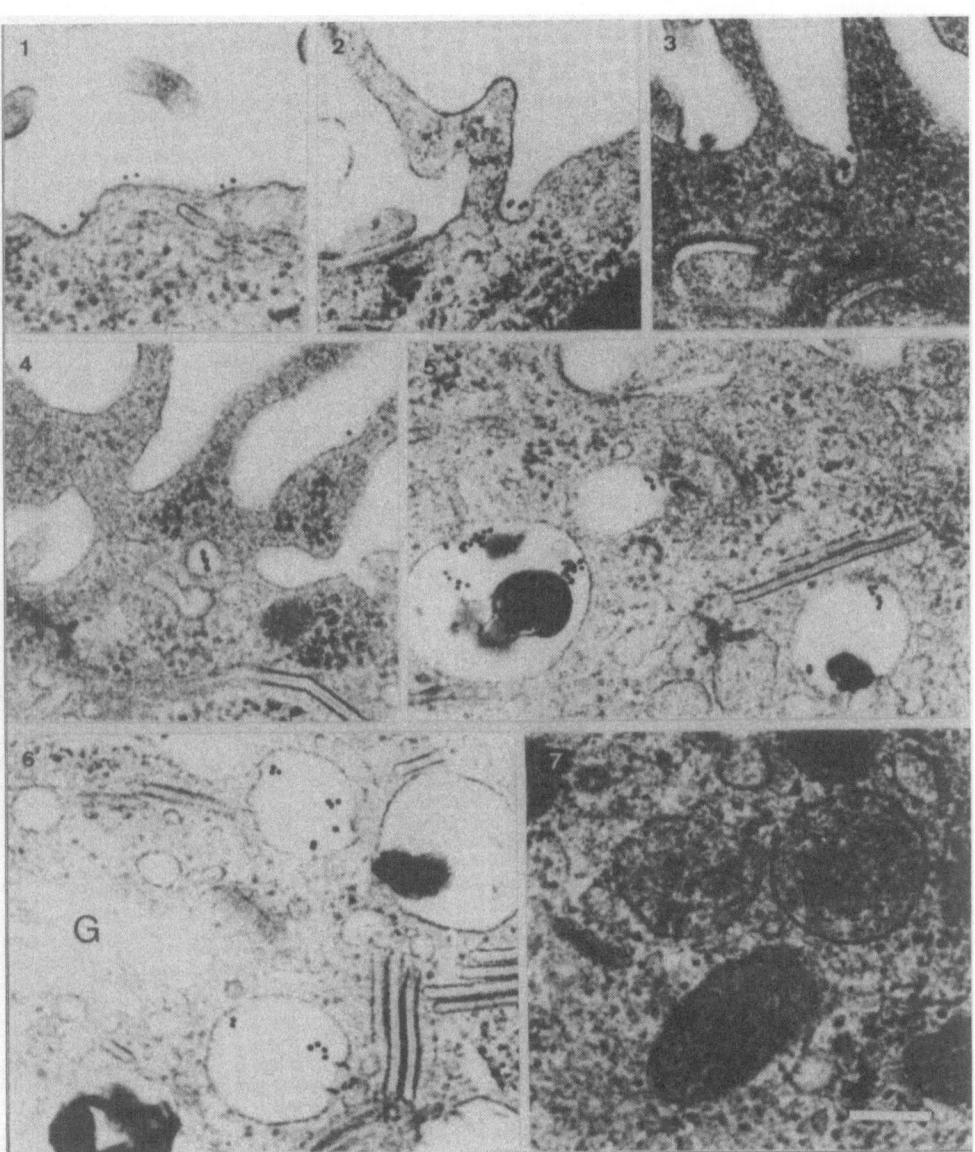

Fig. 11.1. Internalization process of the envelope glycoprotein (gp120) by epidermal Langerhans cells. Epidermal LC are successively incubated for one hour at 4°C with 15 nm-labeled gp120 (15 nm-gp120) and for 5, 30 and 60 minutes at 37°C. The envelope proteins (15 nm-gp120) moderately bind to the cell membrane (1). After 5 minutes at 37°C, the 15 nm-gp120 is internalized through receptor-mediated endocytosis, gold granules are found in coated pits and coated vesicles (2-4). After 30 minutes at 37°C, gold particles are found in intracytoplasmic organelles, i.e. endosomes (5, 6) and lysosomes (7). (G = Golgi apparatus, bar = 200 nm).

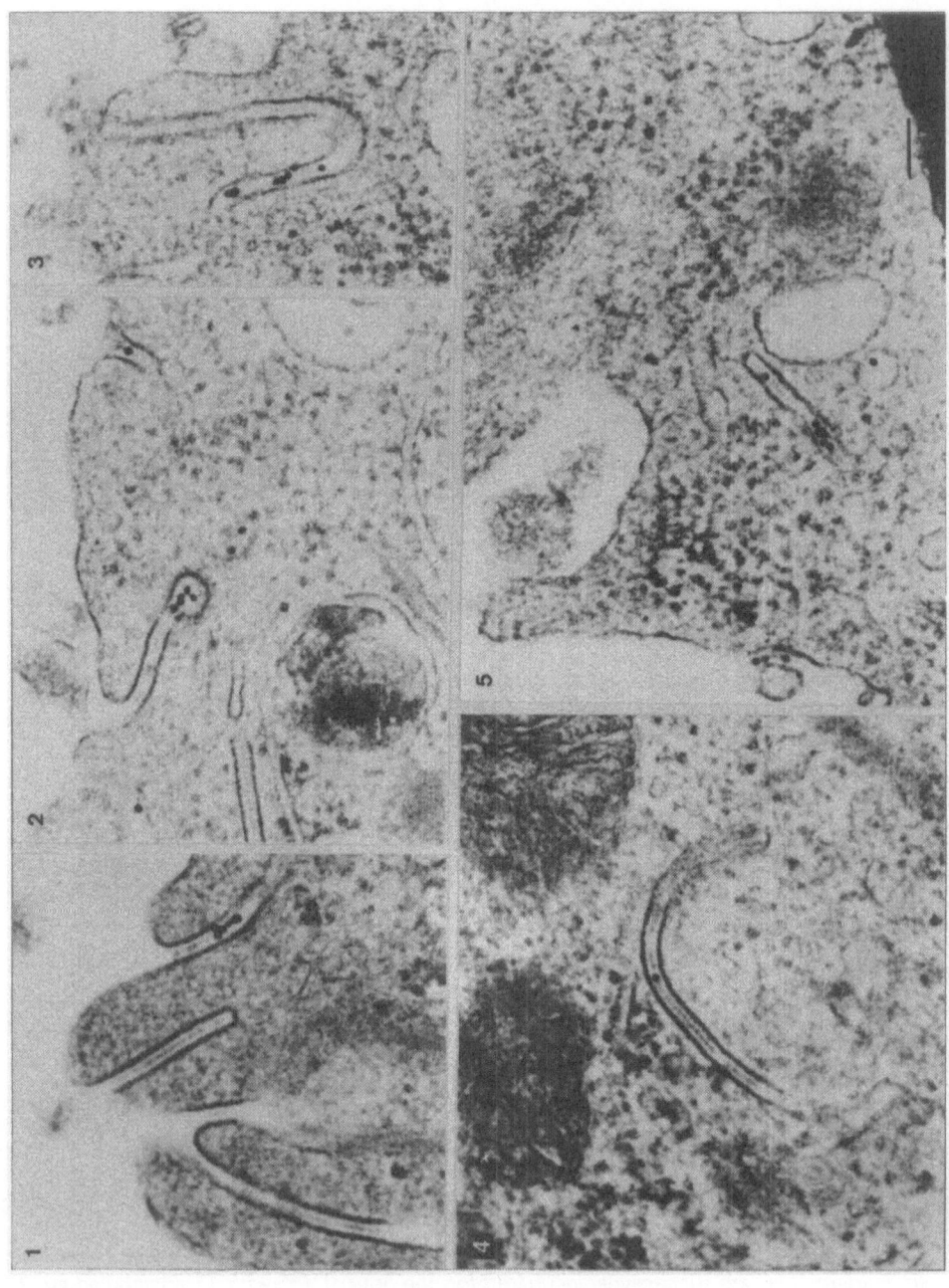

Fig. 11.2. Internalization process of the envelope glycoprotein (gp120) by epidermal Langerhans cells. The 15 nm-gp120 is also internalized through Birbeck granules which are generated from the plasma membrane of LC (1-3), progressively detached from the membrane and are found in the cytoplasm (4, 5). (Bar = 200 nm).

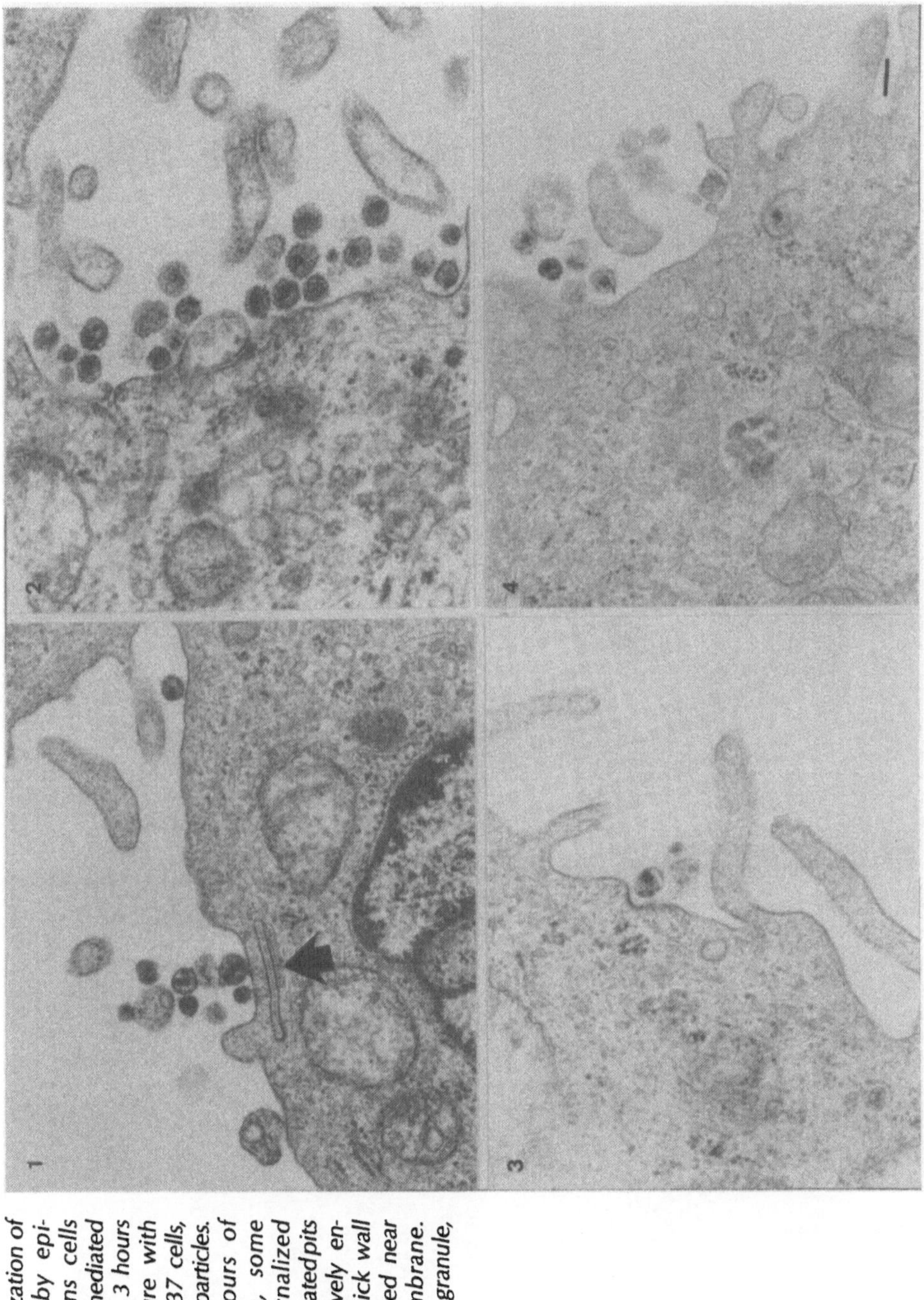

Fig. 11.3. Internalization of HIV-1 particles by epidermal Langerhans cells through receptor-mediated endocytosis. After 3 hours (1, 2) of coculture with HIV-1-carrying U937 cells, LC tightly bind viral particles. Then, after 6 hours of coculture (3, 4), some virions are internalized through clathrin-coated pits (3) and progressively enclosed in small thick wall vesicles (4) localized near the plasma membrane. (Arrow = Birbeck granule, bar = 100 nm).

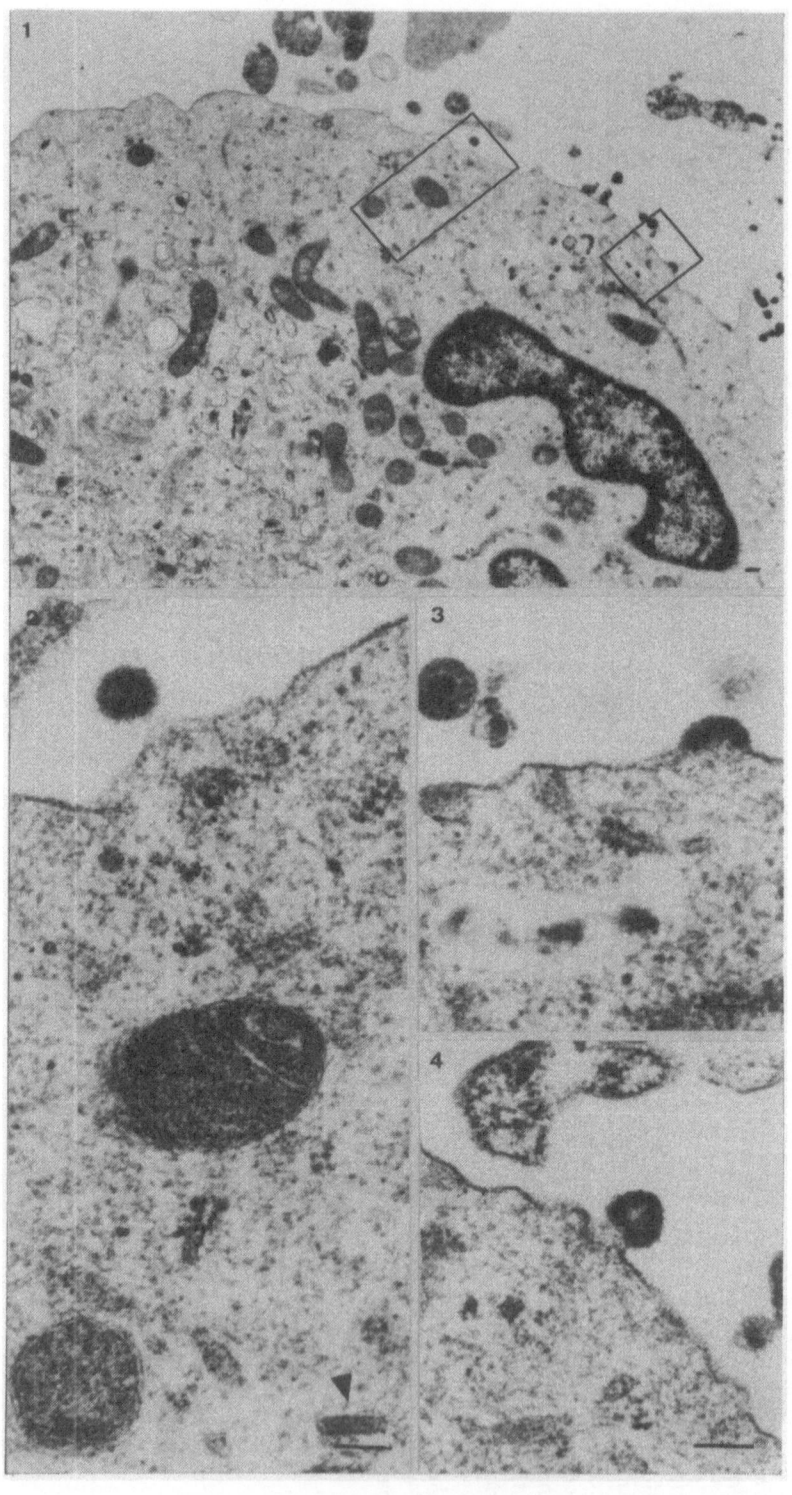

filtration. Proviral DNA (*gag* gene sequences) was found in LC-enriched epidermal cellular DNA from day four of infection with the HIV-IIIB isolate and from day seven with HIV-RF isolate. Although the reverse transcriptase activity did not reach a significantly high level, viral RNA could be determined in supernatant of LC-enriched epidermal cell cultures at the time when proviral DNA was detected. These last findings indicate that the cell-free virus infection model leads to a later-occurring infection and a lower HIV expression than does cell-to-cell transmission. Nevertheless, this model allowed us to confirm the CD4-independent infection of isolated trypsin-treated LC and thus may be attractive for in vitro study of this type of infection. This mode of infection may be ideal to investigate the effectiveness of soluble factors on the mechanism of infection although, among the variety of mechanisms of infection, LC infection through contact-mediated transmission continues to merit consideration.

CONTRIBUTION OF THE FELINE LANGERHANS CELLS TO FIV MUCOSAL TRANSMISSION

Despite the fact that heterosexual contact is the predominant route of transmission, the biology of the heterosexual transmission of HIV remains poorly understood. Mucosal transmission of feline immunodeficiency virus (FIV) in cats under experimental conditions would constitute a valuable model for the heterosexual transmission of HIV. Several difficulties in comparing the HIV and FIV systems lie in the reproductive anatomy and physiology of the cat.[26] In 1987, Pedersen[27] isolated in cats a new retrovirus very similar to HIV, FIV. This virus was detected in saliva, and it is now assumed that bites are the major route of FIV transmission in nature.[28] Furthermore, it was recently demonstrated that FIV transmission may occur through the oral, vaginal and rectal mucous membranes,[29] leading to systemic infection.

We tried to identify the equivalent of human LC in skin and mucous membranes and to find out whether these cells could be a target for FIV in order to demonstrate the contribution of feline

---

Fig. 11.4 (opposite). In vitro infection of isolated epidermal Langerhans cells with a system of coculture. The permissiveness to replication of HIV-1 by LC can be shown by electron microscopy (1). Formation of buds from plasma membrane (3) and release of mature virions are progressively followed (2, 4). (Arrow = Birbeck granules, bar = 100 nm).

LC as an experimental model for the transmission of virus through the mucous membranes. CD18-positive dendritic epithelial cells were found in all epidermal locations and in the mucous membranes (oral, vaginal, rectal and esophageal membranes).[30] Furthermore, these cells presented morphological and ultrastructural characteristics (Birbeck granules) which favor the hypothesis that these CD18-positive cells in cat stratified epithelia are the equivalent of human LC. This observation makes the feline LC a good candidate for an FIV model for exploring the infection of human LC located in the mucous membranes in the initial viral inoculation process.

WHAT COULD BE THE CONSEQUENCES OF HIV/LANGERHANS CELL INTERACTIONS IN VIVO?

The fact that LC seem to support replication of HIV in vitro suggests that these cells may play an important part in viral pathogenesis. The persistence of HIV-producing LC may favor a systemic dissemination of the virus from the areas of inoculation to regional lymph nodes, where infected LC could serve as a constant source of infection for CD4+ T lymphocytes. Nevertheless, the rare demonstration of viral proteins in the epidermal compartment suggests that, in vivo, either infected LC are already migrating from epidermis to lymph nodes or the infected LC are still present in the epidermis with the virus in a latent form. A variety of inducers (viral infections[31,32] and ultraviolet irradiation[33]) may break this latency leading to a reactivation of the virus and subsequent replication.

LC in genital mucosa might also play a role in the initial viral inoculation. LC are abundant in the vaginal and ectocervical mucosa of women and dendritic processes extend to the lumen of the vagina.[34,35] It seems that HIV may first infect LC in the vagina. The infected LC may migrate to draining lymph nodes and interact with CD4+ T lymphocytes. Such an interaction could allow the virus to spread to a large number of cells. Consequently, it is easy to hypothesize a putative role for LC as a vector for dissemination, although the consequences resulting from such an infection on their antigen-presenting cell functions are still not fully explored. The persistence of HIV in LC could alter the antigen-presenting function as it does in monocytes[36] and in dendritic cells[37,38] in the peripheral blood, although this last point seems to be a source of controversy.[39] Nevertheless, any alteration of the immune defense of the skin or mucous membrane environment would amplify the state of immunosuppression characteristic of the HIV infection and make the organism more vulnerable to new infections.

CONCLUSION

Human LC can be considered as targets for HIV infection. HIV-1 proviral DNA is detected in LC from AIDS patients and epidermal LC isolated from normal skin can be infected in vitro with HIV-1. Such experimental infections represent powerful approaches to understanding the regulation of HIV infection of LC. The sites of LC infection have not been clearly established. Such an infection may occur either in LC precursors (found in bone marrow, peripheral blood and dermis) or in mature LC in squamous epithelia. Investigation of the putative infectability of LC precursors generated in vitro in the presence of granulocyte/macrophage colony-stimulating factor (GM-CSF) and tumor necrosis factor α (TNF-α)[40] may provide crucial information on the infection of LC found at different stages of differentiation. HIV transmission by sexual contact would lead to a direct infection of LC in mucosa. In addition, infected LC may constitute a source of HIV infection and transmit virus to T lymphocytes in dermis as well as in peripheral lymph nodes where LC migrate following antigenic stimulation. A better understanding of the basic interactions between LC and HIV may provide insight into rational approaches to preventing infection.

REFERENCES

1. Belsito DV, Sanchez MR, Baer RL et al. Reduced Langerhans cell Ia antigen and ATPase activity in patients with the acquired immunodeficiency syndrome. N Engl J Med 1984; 310:1279-82.
2. Daniels TE, Greenspan D, Greenspan JS et al. Absence of Langerhans cells in oral hairy leukoplasia, an AIDS-associated lesion. J Invest Dermatol 1987; 89:178-82.
3. Dreno B, Milpied B, Bignon J et al. Prognostic value of Langerhans cells in the epidermis of HIV patients. Brit J Dermatol 1988; 118:481-6.
4. Tschachler E, Groh V, Popovic M et al. Epidermal Langerhans cells—A target for HTLV-IIIB/LAV infection. J Invest Dermatol 1987; 88:233-7.
5. Rappersberger K, Gartner S, Schenk P et al. Langerhans cells are an actual site of HIV-1 replication. Intervirology 1988; 29:185-94.

6. Gielen V, Schmitt D, Dezutter-Dambuyant C et al. AIDS and Langerhans cells: CD4 antigenic site density modification evidenced by single-cell immunogold labeling. Reg Immunol 1989; 2:7-13.

7. Berger R, Gartner S, Foster C et al. Langerhans cells infected with HIV-1, in vivo and in vitro, can transmit virus to other hematopoietic cells. J Invest Dermatol 1988; 90:546-51.

8. Kanitakis J, Marchand C, Su H et al. Immunohistochemical study of normal skin of HIV-1-infected patients shows no evidence of infection of epidermal Langerhans cells by HIV. AIDS Res and Human Retrovirus 1989; 5:293-302.

9. Vogel J, Cepeda M, Tschachler E et al. UV activation of human immunodeficiency virus gene expression in transgenic mice. J Virol 1992; 66:1-5.

10. Morrey JD, Bourn SM, Bunch TD et al. In vivo activation of human immunodeficiency virus type 1 long terminal repeat by UV type-A (UV-A) light plus psoralen and UV-B light in skin of transgenic mice. J Virol 1991; 65:5045-51.

11. Morrey JD, Jackson MK, Bunch TD et al. Activation of the human immunodeficiency virus type 1 long terminal repeat by skin-sensitizing chemicals in transgenic mice. Intervirology 1993; 36:65-70.

12. Kanitakis J, Escaich S, Trepo C et al. Detection of human immunodeficiency virus-DNA and RNA in the skin of HIV-infected patients using the polymerase chain reaction. J Invest Dermatol 1991; 97:91-6.

13. Naher H, Schule T, Petzoldt D. Evidence for genetic HIV variants from detection of HIV-DNA. Lancet 1991; 338:519-20.

14. Zambruno G, Mori L, Marconi A et al. Detection of HIV-1 in epidermal Langerhans cells of HIV-infected patients using the polymerase chain reaction. J Invest Dermatol 1991; 96:979-82.

15. Dusserre N, Dezutter-Dambuyant C, Mallet F et al. The in vitro HIV-1 entry and replication in Langerhans cells may clarify the HIV-1 genome detection by PCR in epidermis of seropositive patients. J Invest Dermatol 1992; 99:99-102.

16. Kalter DC, Greenhouse JJ, Orenstein JM et al. Epidermal Langerhans cells are not principal reservoirs of virus in HIV disease. J Immunol 1991; 146:3396-404.

17. Gianetti A, Zambruno G, Cimarelli A et al. Direct detection of HIV-1 RNA in epidermal Langerhans cells of HIV-infected patients. J Acq Immune Def Synd 1993; 6:329-33.

18. Cimarelli A, Zambruno G, Marconi A et al. Quantitation by competitive PCR of HIV-1 proviral DNA in epidermal Langerhans cells of HIV-infected patients. J Acq Immune Def Synd 1994; 7:230-5.

19. Berger R, Gartner S, Rappersberger K et al. Isolation of human immunodeficiency virus type-1 from human epidermis: virus replication and transmission studies. J Invest Dermatol 1992; 99:271-7.

20. Dezutter-Dambuyant C, Schmitt DA, Dusserre N et al. Interac-

tion of human epidermal Langerhans cells with HIV-1 viral envelope proteins (gp 120 and gp 160s) involves a receptor-mediated
endocytosis independent of the CD4 T4A epitope. J Dermatol
1991; 18:377-92.

21. Dezutter-Dambuyant C, Schmitt DA, Dusserre N et al. Trypsin-
resistant gp 120 receptors are upregulated on short-term cultured
human epidermal Langerhans cells. Res Virol 1991; 142:129-38.

22. Braathen LR, Ramirez G, Kunze ROF et al. Langerhans cells in
mucous membrane and skin may be the primary target cells for
HIV. In: Thivolet J, Schmitt D, eds. The Langerhans cells. Libbey
Eurotext 1988; 172:441-8.

23. Dusserre N, Delorme P, Dezutter-Dambuyant C et al. In vitro
transmission of human immunodeficiency virus type-1 from monocytes to epidermal Langerhans cells results in virion entry through
receptor-mediated endocytosis. Europ J Dermatol 1991; 1:139-43.

24. Delorme P, Dezutter-Dambuyant C, Ebersold A et al. In vitro infection of epidermal Langerhans cells with human immunodeficiency
virus type 1 (HTLV-IIIB isolate). Res Virol 1993; 144:53-8.

25. Charbonnier AS, Mallet F, Fiers MM et al. Detection of HIV-
specific DNA sequences in epidermal Langerhans cells infected in
vitro by means of a cell-free system. Arch Dermatol Res 1994; in
press.

26. Miller CJ. Animal models of viral sexually transmitted diseases.
AJRA 1994; 31:52-63.

27. Pedersen NC, Ho EW, Brown ML et al. Isolation of a T-
lymphotropic virus from domestic cats with an immunodeficiency-
like syndrome. Science 1987; 235:790-93.

28. Yamamoto JK, Sparger E, Ho EW et al. Pathogenesis of experimentally induced feline immunodeficiency virus infection in cats.
Am J Vet Res 1988; 49:1246-58.

29. Moench TR, Whaley KJ, Mandrell TD et al. The cat/FIV model
for transmucousal transmission of AIDS: nonoxynol-9 contracep-
tive jelly blocks transmission by an infected cell inoculum. AIDS
1993; 7:797-802.

30. Tsagarakis T, Marchal JP, Magnol C et al. Contribution of the
feline Langerhans cell in the FIV model. Res Virol 1994; 145:245-9.

31. Mosca JD, Bednarik DP, Raj NBK. Herpes simplex virus type-1
can reactivate transcription of latent human immunodeficiency virus. Nature 1987; 325:67-70.

32. Heng MCY, Heng SY, Allen SG. Co-infection and synergy of human immunodeficiency virus-1 and herpes simplex virus-1. Lancet
1994; 343:255-8.

33. Stein B, Kramer M, Rahmsdorf HJ et al. UV-induced transcription from the human immunodeficiency virus type-1 (HIV-1) long
terminal repeat and UV-induced secretion of an extracellular factor
that induced HIV-1 transcription in nonirradiated cells. J Virol
1989; 63:4540-4.

34. Edwards JNT, Morris HB. Langerhans cells and lymphocyte sub-
    sets in the female genital tract. Br J Obstet Gynecol 1985;
    92:974-82.
35. Bjercke S, Scott H, Braathen LR et al. HLA-DR-expressing Langer-
    hans-like cells in vaginal and cervical epithelium. Acta Obstet
    Gynecol Scand 1983; 62:585-9.
36. Rich EA, Toossi Z, Fujiwara H et al. Defective accessory function
    of monocytes in human immunodeficiency virus-related disease syn-
    dromes. J Lab Clin Med 1988; 112:174-81.
37. Macatonia SE, Patterson S, Knight SC. Suppression of immune
    responses by dendritic cells infected with HIV. Immunology 1989;
    67:285-99.
38. Macatonia SE, Gompels M, Pinching AJ et al. Antigen presenta-
    tion by macrophages but not by dendritic cells in human immu-
    nodeficiency virus (HIV) infection. Immunology 1992; 75:576-81.
39. Cameron PU, Forsum U, Teppler H et al. During HIV-1 infec-
    tion most blood dendritic cells are not productively infected and
    can induce allogeneic CD4$^+$ T cells clonal expansion. Clin Exp
    Immunol 1992; 88:226-36.
40. Caux C, Dezutter-Dambuyant C, Schmitt D et al. GM-CSF and
    TNFα cooperate for the generation of dendritic cells: Langerhans
    cells from human hematopoietic progenitors. Nature 1992;
    360:258-61.

INDEX

Page numbers in italics denote figures (f) or tables (t).

MOLECULAR BIOLOGY
INTELLIGENCE UNIT

AVAILABLE AND UPCOMING TITLES

NEUROSCIENCE INTELLIGENCE UNIT

AVAILABLE AND UPCOMING TITLES

MEDICAL INTELLIGENCE UNIT

AVAILABLE AND UPCOMING TITLES

- ☐ Hyperacute Xenograft Rejection
  Jeffrey Platt, Duke University
- ☐ Chimerism and Tolerance
  Suzanne Ildstad, University of Pittsburgh
- ☐ Birth Control Vaccines
  G.P. Talwar and Raj Raghupathy, National Institute of Immunology-New Delhi and University of Kuwait
- ☐ Monoclonal Antibodies in Transplantation
  Lucienne Chatenoud, Hôpital Necker-Paris
- ☐ Therapeutic Applications of Oligonucleotides
  Stanley Crooke, ISIS Pharmaceuticals
- ☐ Cryopreserved Venous Allografts
  Kelvin G.M. Brockbank, CryoLife, Inc.
- ☐ Clinical Benefits of Leukodepleted Blood Products
  Joseph Sweeney and Andrew Heaton, Miriam and Roger Williams Hospitals-Providence and Irwin Memorial Blood Center-San Francisco
- ☐ Delta Hepatitis Virus
  M. Dinter-Gottlieb, Drexel University
- ☐ Intima Formation in Blood Vessels: Spontaneous and Induced
  Mark M. Kockx, Algemeen Ziekenhuis Middelheim-Antwerpen
- ☐ Adult T Cell Leukemia and Related Diseases
  Takashi Uchiyama and Jungi Yodoi, University of Kyoto
- ☐ Development of Epstein-Barr Virus Vaccines
  Andrew Morgan, University of Bristol
- ☐ p53 Suppressor Gene
  Tapas Mukhopadhyay, Steven Maxwell and Jack A. Roth, University of Texas-MD Anderson Cancer Center
- ☐ Sudden Death in Ischemic Heart Disease
  Malcolm D. Silver and Giorgio Baroldi, University of Toronto and University of Milan
- ☐ Minor Histocompatibility Antigens and Transplantation
  Craig V. Smith, University of Pittsburgh
- ☐ Familial Adenomatous Polyposis Coli and the APC Gene
  Joanna Groden, University of Cincinnati
- ☐ Cancer Cell Adhesion and Tumor Invasion
  Pnina Brodt, McGill University
- ☐ Constitutional Immunity to Infection
  Cees M. Verduin, David A. Watson, Jan Verhoef, Hans Van Dijk, University of Utrecht and North Dakota State University
- ☐ Nutritional and Metabolic Support in Critically Ill Patients
  Rifat Latifi and Stanley Dudrick, Yale University
- ☐ Nutritional Support in Gastrointestinal Failure
  Rifat Latifi and Stanley Dudrick, Yale University
- ☐ Septic Myocardiopathy: Molecular Mechanisms
  Karl Werdan, Ludwig-Maximilians-Universität-München
- ☐ The Molecular Genetics of Wilms Tumor
  Max Coppes, Christine Campbell and Bryan R.G. Williams, Cleveland Clinic and University of Calgary
- ☐ Endothelins
  David J. Webb and Gillian Gray, University of Edinburgh
- ☐ Nutritional and Metabolic Support in Cancer, Transplant and Immunocompromised Patients
  Rifat Latifi, Yale University
- ☐ Antibody-Mediated Graft Rejection
  J. Andrew Bradley and Eleanor Bolton, University of Glasgow
- ☐ Liposomes in Cancer Chemotherapy
  Steven Sugarman, University of Texas-MD Anderson
- ☐ Molecular Basis of Human Hypertension
  Florent Soubrier, Collége de France-Paris
- ☐ Endocardial Endothelium: Control of Cardiac Performance
  Stanislas U. Sys and Dirk Brutsaert, Universiteit Antwerpen
- ☐ Endovascular Stented Grafts for the Treatment of Vascular Diseases
  Michael L. Marin, Frank J. Veith and Barry A. Levine, Albert Einstein College of Medicine
- ☐ B Cells and Autoimmunity
  Christian Boitard, Hôpital Necker-Paris
- ☐ Immunity to Mycobacteria
  Ian Orme, Colorado State University
- ☐ Hepatic Stem Cells and the Origin of Hepatic Carcinoma
  Stewart Sell, University of Texas-Houston
- ☐ HLA and Maternal-Fetal Recognition
  Joan S. Hunt, University of Kansas
- ☐ Transplantation Tolerance
  J. Wesley Alexander, University of Cincinnati
- ☐ Ovarian Autoimmunity
  Roy Moncayo and Helga E. Moncayo, University of Innsbruck
- ☐ Ex Vivo Cell Therapy for Cancer
  Ronald Herberman, University of Pittsburgh
- ☐ Protein and Amino Acid Metabolism in Cancer
  Peter W.T. Pisters and Murray Brennan, Sloan-Kettering Memorial Cancer Center
- ☐ Cytokines and Hemorrhagic Shock
  Eric J. DeMaria, Medical College of Virginia
- ☐ Endometriosis
  Lisa Barrie Schwartz, New York University and David Olive, Yale University
- ☐ T Cell Vaccination and Autoimmune Disease
  Jingwu Zhang, Willems Institut-Belgium
- ☐ Immune Privilege
  J. Wayne Streilein, Luke Jiang and Bruce Ksander, Schepens Eye Research Institute-Boston
- ☐ The Pathophysiology of Sepsis and Multi-Organ Failure
  Mitchell Fink, Harvard University
- ☐ Bone Metastasis
  F. William Orr, McMaster University
- ☐ Novel Regional Therapies for Liver Tumors
  Seiji Kawasaki and Masatoshi Makuuchi, Shinshu University
- ☐ Thyroid Hormone Resistance
  Roy E. Weiss and Michael Refetoff, University of Chicago
- ☐ Growth Hormone in Critical Illness
  Michael Torosian, University of Pennsylvania
- ☐ Molecular Biology of Aneurysms
  Richard R. Keen, Northwestern University
- ☐ Strategies in Malaria Vaccine Design
  F.E.G. Cox, King's College London
- ☐ Chimeric Proteins and Fibrinolysis
  Christoph Bode, Marschall Runge and Edgar Haber, University of Heidelberg, University of Texas-Galveston and Harvard University